The Story Addict

The Story Addict

Kjell Benson MD

The Brookbank Press

ISBN: 978-0-9637672-8-8

For my children, Noah, Ephraim and Zella,
so they know what I do all day.

Acknowledgements

First, thanks to all my patients over the years. Thank you for the trust to let me into your lives, and the hope that I would do something to help you. Your lives have given mine meaning, and I hope this book pays tribute to the beauty of your lives. I have changed the names, places and circumstances of the people I have encountered for privacy, but I hope that everyone finds a little of themselves recounted here.

Thanks to my mother Nancy who taught me to write, cultivated a love of reading, led by example in showing that a life serving others is one worth living, and inspired me to write these stories. Thanks to my old friend Hong Mei who tirelessly encouraged me to keep writing and complete the project. Also thanks to friends and family who read drafts and gave comments: Brian Gollnick, Lance Rhoades, Laurie Parker, Marian Rhys.

Finally, thanks to Providence Health which took a chance on sponsoring an unproven new program, just because it was the right thing to do for patients.

Contents

Introduction

"The assumption... has been that the physical place, the actual place, is of no more consequence than the scenery behind a group of actors, something to keep the narrative going while imported ideas unfold against a backdrop." -- Barry Lopez, Horizon

Modern medicine is undergoing an existential crisis. Here on the freeway of unlimited biochemical discoveries, our reach has exceeded our grasp, and we are accumulating more problems than solutions: a widening burden of disease between rich and poor, the public's loss of trust in doctors, physician burnout and even suicide, and a ruinous financial price for the whole system. This book chronicles a tentative step toward a different medical future: home visits that upend the traditional hierarchy of medical expertise and attempt to put the human first, rather than diseases.

In every culture around the world, the home visit has traditionally been the foundation of the healer's craft, and by recreating that dynamic, we may be tapping in to something fundamental. The construction of our modern medical infrastructure, with its hospitals, clinics, pharmacies and always more buildings, has fueled amazing technical discoveries and life-saving treatments, but also diminished the patient as a person. Home visits re-establish the priority of a person, situated in their community and context -- the place we all long to be.

The home is where people cope with illness, day after day, so visiting it engages a humanitarian aspect of healthcare. This humanism is often lost in healthcare's endless buildings, but is also usually why providers went in to the field of medicine in the first place. These stories relate my own journey to humanism in medicine, through my training, the books I read, and the patients I try to help. Everyone in medicine makes this journey, navigating between the art and the science, arriving somewhere where they can use science as a tool rather than a bludgeon.

My journey documented in these stories involves the slow realization of how too much medical care harms rather than helps, how my disabled son has given me wisdom and empathy, and how stories, the sea of stories, sustain us all. Home is where the health is. And it may be the beginning of a rebirth of modern medicine.

Are You a Frail, Complex Patient?

"The end of our foundation is the knowledge of causes, and secret motions of things; and the enlarging of the bounds of human empire, to the effecting of all things possible". -- Francis Bacon, *New Atlantis*

Michael recently retired from a long career as a clothing store owner in one of the growing communities surrounding Portland, Oregon. He was vigorous, and worked incessantly to run a small business in a competitive market. "I had a good run," he said. "I retired 18 months ago..."

His wife interrupts, "You did not retire, that's the whole problem."

"So, I retired and sold the business, but can you believe some people? The guy could not run a business, he just wrecked it!" He pauses.

"Go on," his wife chimes in again, "tell him what you did then."

"I had to fix it! I guess I un-retired again for a while... But now I have been retired again for 4 months. This time for good."

They own a house, and some surrounding property, with a view of the hills. Lush, verdant, and he now had upgraded from a push mower to a John Deere sitting model. This is a Portland paradise.

Today is his initial visit with our program, and he brings me into the dining nook so we can sit at the table and talk. "Oh, honey, you have to let me explain stuff," he tells his wife as she starts into all the symptoms that bother him. We spend 15 minutes reviewing what our home visit program is and is not, and what he can expect.

"We will try to impact your life by coordinating the care of your various specialists. Sometimes it can be tricky to negotiate our system, I know that." He nods his head as I explain. "We also will be able to spend more time with you than other doctors often can. For example, today I have an hour here with you. And then we see if we can reduce the amount of medicines and tests by only focusing on the most efficient and useful ones. And finally, we are available by phone 24 hours a day if something comes up where you need help. If needed, we can even come out here to your house -- I have IVs, and medications, and a full clinic in the back of my car."

I am thinking I would not mind being called out here. I am sitting at the round table with a checked cloth and looking out the window to a field with a horse grazing and a forested hill in the background. Peace. I have to pull my attention back to Michael as he eagerly launches into his medical saga.

"I am tired all the time. I don't sleep well. My knees hurt. My urologist wants to do another procedure on my bladder and I'm not sure if I should or not. I am so tired of just eating salads, and it doesn't seem to matter with my blood sugar anyway. I can't work in my shop anymore. Sometimes I just sleep out there on the couch instead. My diabetes doctor retired and I am supposed to go all the way across town to some specialist, but what for? They just give me another pill..."

Out pours a jumble of symptoms, diseases and frustrations. It is actually surprisingly easy to answer the question of whether you are frail and complex medically: are you defined by your medical conditions, or do you define your own medical care? People with simple, discrete illnesses are able to effectively manage their own treatments, by making appointments, following recommendations and evaluating experts' advice to arrive at the best course of action. Those we define as "medically complex" can no longer effectively achieve any of these goals on their own. With five chronic conditions, more than eight medications, a primary care provider and multiple specialists, making sense of all the advice becomes daunting. Michael has "after-visit summaries" from two hospitals and three clinics, all sitting tucked into a folder. They contain contradictory advice and medication lists that don't match.

Michael has diabetes which is poorly controlled and requires 100 units of insulin injected twice daily. He has overactive bladder, which means out of the blue, his bladder muscle contracts randomly, causing him to feel that he has to urinate, so he runs to the bathroom, sometimes making it in time, sometimes not. He admits to being "stressed" all the time, tried some antidepressant medications for a short time but it worsened his sleep and he quit. He had a renal cell cancer ten years ago, treated very effectively by surgery to "remove half my kidney". And he thinks at one point he had chest pain and he went to a doctor who told him that he had had a heart attack. He thinks his primary care doctor is good, but does not like to go because she just asks a few questions and then changes a pill and says, "I'll see you in three months..." I'm not sure we are going to be able to cover all this even with an hour visit.

New doctors who take on complex home-based care tend to repeat the mistake that all Michael's specialists are making, focusing on one disease and trying to improve it. Of course, these diseases work together, in a motley interrelated system called the human body. Increasing his insulin might lower blood sugars a little, but the small syringe full of insulin, when increased about 50 units, becomes a large syringe full of liquid injected into tissue below the skin. It is possible to do, but when you have a few milliliters of fluid injected and just sitting there in a glob, does it get absorbed into the bloodstream? How quickly? How does that affect the blood sugars? So then we have to use a super-concentrated insulin to decrease the volume of liquid injected... It gets complicated. Instead we need to take a step back and try to find patterns between the diseases that will allow synergies of therapies, and a reduction of complexity rather than an increase.

Obstructive sleep apnea has become a modern epidemic due primarily to the concurrent rise of obesity. The human airway is a fragile tube-like passage from the back of the throat down to the larynx and then the bronchus into the lungs. It serves triple duty, transporting air, allowing speech, and transporting and diverting food away from the lungs to the stomach. With obesity, the soft tissues surrounding the airway become swollen, and with sleep, the muscles holding the airway open relax. The airway closes and people stop breathing, but don't realize it because they are sleeping. Eventually, within 30 seconds or so, the blood oxygen level falls, the carbon dioxide level rises, and the primitive brainstem, the "animal brain" sends a signal to the higher brain to wake up and breathe. So the person awakens, partially, restoring muscle tone, opening the airway and taking a breath, restoring the oxygen level. Soon sleep recurs, and the cycle repeats. Unfortunately, each time the brain signals to awaken, it also sends a surge of panic hormones like adrenaline. So with sleep apnea, the body is subjected to hundreds of surges of adrenaline each night as it constantly re-awakens itself. Adrenaline raises blood sugar levels, it raises blood pressure, it strains the heart. In short it messes with the whole body, fine once in a while on a roller coaster, but not healthy when it occurs all the time.

We have to start by somehow getting a handle on Michael's sleep apnea. This will allow him to actually rest. It will lower his blood sugars without more insulin. It will ease the strain on the heart. It will allow him to be more active during the day, which will improve diabetes and his diet, etc. But he had a bad experience at the sleep lab where they did the sleep apnea testing. He never wants to go back.

Nobody said this was going to be simple. "Tell me more about your sleep," I begin.

Heroin is the Sickness Unto Death

"In despairing over something, he really despaired over himself, and now he wants to be rid of himself." --Soren Kierkegaard, The Sickness Unto Death

Sara has cafe-au-lait skin and dark hair. Her eyes are darker still, retreating back and yet farther back from her face, fleeing. She cannot sit still, and twists amongst the bedsheets, caught. Her clothes are used, terribly used, to the point of fraying into their original uncolored color: grey. She is a person trapped in a body. As I counsel her regarding the diagnosis of an infected heart valve, I notice she is staring out the window.

She arrived in the emergency department gasping for breath, with fevers, chills, and arms tattooed with needle tracks. Dirty needles, dirty dope, and repeated exposures means that every addict will eventually seed themselves with deadly bacteria into the bloodstream. And those bacteria eventually settle on the heart valves, growing and multiplying despite the body's attempts to fight them. Sepsis, with bacterial seed pods flicked out from the heart on every beat, taking the superhighway to internal organs. Mild skin infections leading to deeper abscesses, infected pockets along the spinal column destroying the bony supports and causing paralysis, heart valves blown open as the connective tissue erodes; infections in the bloodstream eventually cause all these and more.

Heroin users are doomed to be addicts. You cannot casually use heroin. The way it short-circuits our free will led to our current epidemic and societal crisis. Strangely, this bypass also opens a window into humans' existential dilemma. My patient listens to a discussion of her imminent death by infected valve and yet stares out the window. Her mind is just not on the subject. If she does not complete six weeks of strong intravenous antibiotics, the infection on the valve will grow, destroy the valve and cause her death as the blood reverses in her heart and backs up into the lungs, filling them with fluid. A gurgling, labored death, shivering under some bridge. I don't sugarcoat the picture saying, "You might die." I always tell them, "You will die. The question is just when." Yet, somehow she cannot focus on this conversation, the most important conversation that anyone could ever have, a plan to maintain your body's existence in this world, and with it the possibility of relationships, pleasure and pain.

My patient's body hurt "all over," but mostly when she took a breath, when the pain radiated to the middle of her upper back. Her left forearm had needle tracks with a palpable corded vein where the poison had clotted and scarred injection sites. There is a wild look in heroin eyes that radiates despair. She cannot contemplate the future. Heroin creates an endless "right now". Without planning for the future, she cannot envision death. And without imagining her death, she is bound to die. Kierkegaard said, "Thus to be sick unto death is to be unable to die, yet not as if there were hope of life; no, the hopelessness is that there is not even the ultimate hope, death."

We know how this story proceeds, for it is a Greek tragedy with its ending foretold before the story even begins. The "heroine" has a fatal flaw. A heart valve infection from dirty needles and dirty drugs -- right sided endocarditis with septic pulmonary emboli. Blood cultures with *Staphylococcus aureus*. Homeless. A "boyfriend" who brings a backpack to her apartment and spends a lot of time in the bathroom. The standard of treatment for this woman would be intravenous antibiotics for weeks; we used to recommend six. But the logistics of that are impossible. How to maintain an

IV line in someone who would rather use it as access for the next high? How to deliver medications at home when there is no home? Various infectious disease studies have experimented with a shorter treatment course, down to even two weeks of IV antibiotics. Even this will be nearly impossible for her to accomplish.

I try to arrange follow up through NARA, the Native American Rehabilitation Association. She has been there, and its motto, Mission Driven, Spirit Led, is what she needs. There is no spirit left in these eyes. “I’ll be ok doc, I just need to go now. I’ve got stuff to do.” There is always stuff to do. There is always something which is not what is happening right now.

What has made America such fertile ground for the poppy and its viral epidemic of opium, heroin and narcotics? We don’t grow it here; it is not “native”. In Afghanistan, where the poppy is grown and harvested, and sold and exported, supporting the economy of otherwise bankrupt peoples, it is not used or abused. The same is true in South America, and in the plentiful poppy fields of Mexico.

My mind also drifts off, to another imported plague. Four hundred years ago smallpox imported from Europe devastated native America. A population with no innate immunity was exposed to something from outside itself, and the results were a disease with no cure, and a culture changed forever. What are the factors that allow the same malady to manifest so differently in different places and different cultures? Why is this continent doomed to suffer from imported plagues? Is there any point to this conversation as my patient stares out the window? Or are we just marionettes, endlessly parroting our roles, me the doctor, she the addict. Seemingly nothing can change her outcome, and similarly seemingly nothing can change my "compassionate" words about her health, the silly endless prattle that doctors learn over years of haranguing patients. Just so, without change, the scene sticks forever in my mind: the tired woman, framed by the window, the needle tracks, my words floating out into the room like cartoon speech balloons. Time is frozen because nothing can change.

Stuck on East Burnside

"Maybe the road could provide a therapy through observation of the ordinary and obvious, a means whereby the outer eye opens an inner one, STOP, LOOK, LISTEN, the old railroad crossing signs warned." – William Least Heat-Moon, Blue Highways

Gridlock on my route from one home visit to another. East 3rd and Burnside. Gas, brake, gas, accelerate. Illness behind, illness ahead. The Portland winter is dark and wet. The gutters glisten from reflected headlights. Not even the water moves fast here, pooling into the low spots, laconically swirling as a tire passes only to settle back with an oily sheen. Abdominal pain was the complaint. The final diagnosis after an hour in the apartment, talking and listening, examining some lab tests: constipation.

The inability to have regular bowel movements has emerged as America's most common invented illness. The mammalian bowel is built to move, constantly. It starts moving before birth and keeps moving until death. Somehow the modern urban human has managed to slow and even stop this inevitable physiological process. The societal cost of our constipated populace is outrageous. I am currently providing home visits for the fragile elderly, trying to help them stay well and out of the hospital. And believe me, constipation can put people straight into intensive care. I have worked everywhere in medicine, from primary care to hospitalist to nursing homes. Constipation gums up the works everywhere, causing pain, then nausea, escalating worry, escalating white blood cell counts, creating abnormal lab tests, all resulting in long and expensive medical examinations and CT scans with the final diagnosis: full of poop.

Martina spends most of the day lying in bed. She lives with her daughter but also qualifies for some "caregiver" time due to disability. She has a paid attendant who spends a few hours daily with her, helping with bathing, chores and other routine tasks that most people take for granted. She calls frequently due to "urinary issues" and abdominal cramps.

“Hi doctor, let’s sit out here so we can talk freely for a moment,” Audra says as she escorts me through the screen door into the living room. Down the corridor lies her mother’s room. The living room looks out onto the yard. Here is where the ubiquitous large television screen sits. Out here is the world of light, action and time. The dark hallway leads to the sealed off room, the timeless universe of illness where her mother exists.

“Sure, we can sit here and talk for a bit, but then I’d like to go spend some time with Martina, so I can hear from her what is going on.” I respond carefully because many families want to carefully orchestrate the doctor’s visit and what I tell to whom. Sometimes this is due to cultural values and the accepted role of the adult child. Sometimes it is simply due to manipulative family dynamics. I am suspicious.

“I think she is getting dementia,” Audra continues. “She is just crazy now, saying stuff. She just makes things up.”

We eventually make our way down the hallway to the back room and see Martina. She lies propped up in bed, queen of her bedchamber. Her daughter Audra and the caregiver hover around from one side to the other, wringing their hands and worrying.

“What does it feel like when you urinate, when you pee?” I steer the conversation away from the fraught issue of dementia to the prosaic of basic functioning.

“Sometimes I have cramps, just along here, and here,” she points to her left and right sides.

There really is no pain in the middle, over the bladder, I discover while examining her abdomen. It had been days since her last bowel movement. Her colon is distended, which then pushes on the bladder and causes irritation. The bladder spasms, urine leaks, the belly is painful, the patient attributes everything to the clear and obvious symptom: the urine. It must be infected. Urinary infections are so common, and she has been “diagnosed” with one many times and given antibiotics. But the symptoms don’t really ever resolve, they just wax and wane. And the reason is that the issue is constipation.

What created the constipation crisis? The opioid epidemic has not helped, as narcotics do slow the bowel, but most people who can’t “go” are not taking morphine. No, the origins of bowel immobility lie in immobility itself. As with most modern chronic diseases, we stopped having bowel movements when we stopped moving. The inactivity of the Western lifestyle is astounding and the consequences inevitable. Never before in history have so many people moved so little. We stare at computers, we drive cars, we take elevators. We operate machinery. From a chair, pulling levers. Kids don’t play outside or run around. Adults don’t walk to work or the store. And the elderly often never even leave their chairs.

Hand in hand with immobility, our society has created processed food. We stopped growing food, harvesting food, and even preparing food. So prepared food appeared, and so we ate fewer fresh foods, with less fiber, and eventually... people don't move, they eat starchy glue-like foods, and a cottage industry of laxatives and consultants was born.

The traffic on Burnside is constipated as well, not moving except in random fits and starts. Traffic was meant to flow, just like the intestines. When it does not, the result is irritation, just as in the colon where I have seen stool impactions create angry, red tissue, cramps, and pain. They have the same ancestry, the constipated bowel and the gridlocked street. The same factors created them: humanity's immobility and poor urban planning. If we walked or cycled to work there would be no jam up. If we had planned smaller urban pockets that preserved agricultural areas, we would have fresh food with fiber to eat rather than endless shrink-wrapped starch.

Humanity suffers from many real maladies that occur due to biological inevitability. Cancer, that most captivating of all diseases, appears to result in a random way from the structure of cell division and DNA storage. Heart disease results from a side-effect of cholesterol which is required for cell membranes. And so on for most human disease. But not constipation. Mammalian evolution never imagined constipation as an issue. As modern hygiene and antibiotics increased the human lifespan, still constipation only rarely occurred. Until we outfoxed ourselves by creating too many modern conveniences, and sank inevitably into the comfortable couch of the 20th century.

Martina and her daughter do not believe me when I say the urine is not infected.

"But I have to go all the time!" she continues to complain.

The distended colon, the thin-walled bladder, the irritation, I repeat my explanation. What is an explanation really? My attempt to give an understandable analogy for underlying scientific principles. It sounds good, but sometimes the "principles" are understood differently by someone who thinks of the bladder as a plastic sack rather than the image I have in my head, the tissue at the end of the scissors during gross anatomy lab dissecting my cadaver as a medical student. Or the image at the end of the videoscope while I assist a urologist doing a flexible video scoping of the bladder during my residency. Or worse, sometimes the ideas I have to convey are simply mathematical conclusions from scientific studies: most post-menopausal women will have bacteria in their urine all the time even though it is not an infection.

Sometimes I can't translate my reality into my patient's terms. Martina is suffering while lying in bed, and her world revolves around this periodic suffering now. My explanations don't touch this fact. The pain pills are sacred and therefore cannot be related to the cramping she has in her belly, to the frequent urination and burning. People create their own stories and I am just a bit player on their stage. Who am I to insist that I am the narrator or have the starring role? I cajole, I bargain, I draw a picture. I sit on the side of the bed and discuss the photos of the grandkids on the dresser. Sometimes we create a story together that involves opioids and constipation, and sometimes I end up prescribing three days of antibiotics for "frequency" caused by a belly full of stool.

I console myself; the doctor is not always right after all. I flick on the turn signal to finally exit this self-inflicted misery of East Burnside. We have met the enemy, and he is us. Medicine is a mix of the banal and the terrifying.

Rocky Butte Record

I had another dream about lions at the door
They weren't half as frightening as they were before
But I'm thinking about eternity
Some kind of ecstasy got ahold of me
-- *Bruce Cockburn*

Dementia: an old woman slowly failing, and no longer eating. I am called to the house because she "does not feel right" and they aren't sure if they should take her to the emergency room. They live on the side of Rocky Butte, one of many old volcanic plugs that poke up out of the plain of East Portland. The developed side of the hill faces west and the golden evening sun streams in. But my patient waits in a back room; perhaps it was once a study, but has now become sanctuary of an old, old woman, fading out of the world surrounded by remnants of her life. She snores peacefully, sitting up in her easy chair, covered with a blanket. They say she is not eating anymore. Does this mean she has some acute intestinal ailment, or is it simply the progression of dementia, which eventually makes the brain forget how to do everything, including eating?

The medical records hold the accounts of a lifetime of interaction with the medical community of Portland. She had heart disease, with its typical "clogged" arteries. She had severe disease in the main artery coming off the aorta which feeds the entire heart. Stents don't work as well in that situation, so she had a coronary artery bypass graft -- CABG, or "cabbage" as the professionals call it. This is a remarkable surgery, perfected over years of practice and communal scientific wisdom. After anesthesia on the operating table, the surgeon uses an electric saw to cut through the breastbone and "crack the chest." Then sturdy retractors pull open the chest cavity, exposing the beating heart. Large tubes pierce the great vessels to divert blood from the heart, run down outside the operating field to a "bypass machine" which takes over for circulating the blood while the heart is stopped. Then, meticulously the surgeon grafts on small veins or arteries harvested from the chest wall or the legs. The stakes are high, as a mistake causes catastrophic bleeding. But the reward is great, because at the end, the heart has new clean arteries piping blood directly from the aorta to the thirsty muscle walls.

After surgery, the breastbone gets sewn up with metal wire and the patient is whisked off to recovery. The post-operative chest x-ray shows the steel wires looped around the sternum and twisted tight. The wire stays in place and shows up on x-rays for the rest of the patient's life, a permanent reminder of a few hours of a scientific miracle. A life is literally saved and a person given back their ability to exercise. But the wires are not the only abiding effects of this miracle. The clamps placed across the aorta crack the calcified walls of the blood vessels and microscopic particles escape into the blood circulation and arrive in other organs. In the brain these microscopic particles appear to slightly alter personalities, and moods. Depression, and worsening cognitive function after these surgeries is common. Sometimes the kidneys are affected and can decline, occasionally even requiring dialysis. Life-long blood thinners are required to prevent the newly grafted arteries from clotting up. The scar tissue can cause fluid to accumulate in the lungs. The manipulation of the heart muscle can make the electrical activity unstable, causing irregular heartbeats, which entail a whole new pathway of diagnosis and treatment. The surgery is miraculous, and its life-changing consequences entail an entire future of ongoing medical care and doctor visits.

Humans are the species defined by modifying themselves. Modern medicine does this to an unprecedented degree. We are slowly creating ourselves anew as a species, and the new human is never simpler than the old. This old woman with the thin scar vertically over her breastbone had started to have memory and confusion issues after her heart surgery. There were various specialist visits where there was concern that she had "vascular dementia", that is decay of brain tissue from many small showers of clots from the heart to the brain such as her "cabbage" might have created. Others thought that she was developing more classic Alzheimers dementia, which does not have such a clear causal agent. There were a lot of doctors' notes. It is a lot of work to take care of a life after it has been saved.

I look around the room after performing a physical examination. There are not many clues to the disease on the body itself so perhaps the more expansive "body", the house and the environment, can help me diagnose. The wall across from the couch is nearly bare, except for a single framed hanging. Not a picture, and I look more closely. Behind the clear glass, with a simple wooden frame, sits a silver phonograph record, cut with a thousand grooves, motionless in the frame but clearly meant to be played. This was a framed vinyl record, with a small photo of a man in uniform in the upper left corner. Dementia cruelly takes away recent memories, but usually preserves more distant life events, and the door into a suffering mind is usually a discussion of the distant past. What is this record on the wall?

She made it for her husband away fighting WWII in the Pacific. He received it but never played it, just framed it to remember her by. What? It has never been played? How did she have it made back in the 40's, in North Dakota? There must have been an expedition to a city with a recording studio. She saved her money, for months, planning her gift. She and a friend took the bus to Minneapolis and found a basement studio where she sang. There was only money for one "take". She missed a note, she halted and froze. Time stopped, but then she picked up again. There was only money for a single try. She gets to the end of the song, the tape stops. Her heart is in her mouth, now so dry after her lyrical verses. Her gift, her savings, is it ruined? Ca...Can I hear it? She quavers. Another take'll cost ya 10 bucks, the gruff man spits out over his dangling cigarette. He has no sympathy; these war brides are at his mercy. They need to make these records and send them. He needs the money. Minneapolis is cold in the winter. Maxine decides not to preview the tape. There is nothing to change. What's done is done. The afternoon is late and the November chill steals into the basement, hurrying her out the door with her friend. They had arranged to stay at the Lutheran church, based on a word from their pastor.

The bus ride back to North Dakota is long. Long and flat. She clutches the brown paper package with a vinyl impressing. Her voice, graven into grooves, one long groove tracing a path from the outside to the inside. Her song for her husband, her husband's song; will she see him again? So many never did and instead have tombstones to visit and a gash rather than a groove.

Now the scene shifts to a destroyer in the South Pacific. The package arrives. Fragile in red letters on the paper covering. The paper peels back, the record emerges, miraculously unbroken. But there is no phonograph on the ship, and they have already left port. There is no room for personal objects on this war mission, each man has only the bunk with a small foot locker. The record does not fit in the locker. How to preserve it? He has the ship's carpenter frame it and they put it on the wall in the mess. It hangs there for the next 9 months until Japan surrenders and he is mustered out. There is a joyful reunion on the Portland docks, and the stockily framed phonograph record has survived both the war and the journey back from the war. But now the couple is reunited and they sing together around the piano. Why unpack an old record to hear a voice which is so much better in person anyway? The record has hung on the wall ever since, perfect behind its glass.

If I could find a phonograph with the right rotation speed, 45? 78 rpm? Those ancient grooves would sing again, I am sure. This woman in front of me is dying; nothing can be done. Her face is peaceful and her eyes closed, a slow fade rather than a violent struggle against the unknown. The moment stretches indefinitely with sun enlarging the room and dedicated son and daughter-in-law collected around her, busy with nondescript household tasks. The record on the wall watches over the scene with a million grooves that reflect the light and an endless story. Its light completes my ritual of packing the blood pressure cuff, and ensuring that the family have the number to call if she appears to be suffering at all. How many lives have been so well captured in a grooved slab of vinyl?

The family asks how long she has. Somehow this is a ritual, I'm sure of it. We go through this call and response every time. Families ask, and I answer with, "No one knows, sometimes more, sometimes less." They press, "I know, you can't say, but just give us your best guess." And on it goes, back and forth. If she has an intestinal obstruction, where the bowel is blocked by a tumor, or a twisting upon itself, the obstructed piece will swell, become more and more painful, then eventually rupture and cause a quick death by septic shock from the gut bacteria seeding the normally sterile abdominal cavity. But this not eating trend is more likely an upset stomach, or just simply no longer having the sensation of hunger. The real question is: if we do more testing, and find colonic cancer obstructing the intestines, would it change what should be done? Would it change what could be done? Would we cut open the belly of this peacefully sleeping woman, remove some pieces, sew her up again and try to get her to heal, when she already refuses food? I don't know when she will die, but I know it should be here in this sun-filled room with the evening light, and not in a sterile hospital room.

Everyone who has encountered Alzheimers dementia understands that their loved one is declining. Everyone knows someone with dementia, has seen the shows, has read the books. However, somewhere the narrative skips off track with the idea that the decline will be "gradual". The decline can be slow, it takes years, but it is rarely gradual. Decline happens with acute events, like an episode of pneumonia, or a stroke, or a hospitalization. What might be an acute illness with a convalescence and recovery for someone more resilient, becomes an abrupt tumble in dementia. The illness gets treated, but the patient has fallen, not off the cliff of mortality, but at least off the stair step on the way there. After the acute issue, recovery just does not occur, the step down cannot be reversed. The decline is irreversible after just a minor event. And then the dementia can plateau for a while, until another acute illness, and another step-off...

"I don't know if this stomach trouble will be the final blow that takes your mother, but I do know that she is falling off a step right now. I just don't know where the bottom of that step will be. I'm sorry."

Tom Has Diarrhea

"Tell me to what you are loyal, and why, -- and you tell me at once just what constitutes the really moral aspect of your personality. All the rest is chance, or fortune, or prejudice or barren routine." -- Josiah Royce, <u>The Philosophy of Loyalty</u>

I get the inevitable phone call, the panicked voice complaining of stomach cramps and sweating. So I go to visit Tom in a small basement apartment across the street from a hospital. He gets unexplained bouts of severe sweating, nausea and diarrhea. The first time we thought this was just a viral "stomach bug" and started an IV in his living room, waiting while the bag infused and his parakeet looked on. But it kept happening. He has gone to the emergency room across the street but complains that they just label him a "drug seeker". Which he might be, actually. He has taken a fair bit of narcotics, and oxycodone dramatically eases the cramping and pain.

As a child, Tom suffered a traumatic brain injury which changed his personality forever. Severe brain injuries to the frontal areas cause people to show their disinhibited mean streaks. Combine that with simplistic black and white thinking, and it was often very challenging to get along with Tom. In a heartbeat, he could interpret what you were saying as a personal attack and turn his flashing eyes and underbite on you, yelling. He had been fired from most medical providers, and he had fired the neighborhood ER staff himself, saying he would "never go back there."

He moans from the couch, "Come in!" as I knock at his low door. I let myself in, familiar with his place by now. Basement apartments should somehow be outlawed in Portland, where the winter light can be so low anyway, but in a north-facing basement, it becomes like living in a movie theater. He has managed to cope on his own as an adult, due to lots of help from various social service agencies. He does his own cooking and shopping, and he spends a lot of time with his parakeet.

"Doc, I'm dying, help me!" He curls in his chair and really does not look too good with a pale face covered in sweat and unkempt hair hiding his eyes. Every few minutes he jumps up to run to the bathroom, and comes back, shaking. Unfortunately, with the sweating, cramping, and questionably dilated pupils, the picture looks a lot like narcotic withdrawal. And when his symptoms ease with IV narcotics, most of health care writes him off as a "druggie". I carry numerous medications around with me, but we made a conscious decision not to carry any narcotics, sort of a "Driver carries no cash" sign. So I can't offer what he really wants, but I can give some IV fluids, and while it trickles into a vein in his arm, we talk.

"How many times have you had episodes like this?" I ask.

"All the time! Stop asking that! Why can't anyone believe me?"

"I believe you, and I need to know a few more details so I can get to the bottom of what is happening. Did these start after your surgery last year?"

Tom had a cancer removed from his abdomen, and it takes me some digging through records to find out that the pathology was not the typical colon adenocarcinoma, but a carcinoid tumor. Carcinoid is a fascinatingly rare cancer that forms from neuroendocrine cells that multiply out of control, and sometimes secrete hormones at high rates. Most cancers form from relatively inert tissue, so the ill effects of the cancer arise only from the bulk effect of cells invading where they should not. Endocrine tumors form from active cells involved in our body's signaling systems, and when they go rogue, they can send huge quantities of strange signals. The pathology report from a year prior indicated that the tumor resection from the small bowel had negative margins and the tumor had been only 2 cm anyways. But the intermittent bouts of sweating, diarrhea and vomiting were classic signs of a carcinoid tumor secreting serotonin and other substances. If this was occurring, Tom had recurrent carcinoid, and was not just withdrawing from narcotics.

For most people, it is not cost-effective to send doctors to their houses for visits. Physicians are expensive, and most office-based medical practices require 20-25 visits per day to break even financially. With home visits, we do only six per day. And yet we still save money for the system because we only take on the most complex patients like Tom. Modern medicine works best when you have a discrete symptom that can be diagnosed as a "disease", and then treated according to a best-practice algorithm. Most people have just such problems: hypertension, ear infections, a broken leg. But as we age, discrete problems become lengthy problem lists, where symptoms overlap and cellular pathology blends into social dysfunction. For these patients, the "system" becomes a quicksand of endlessly more doctors, visits and tests. Tom had fallen into this morass with his quick temper, questionable narcotics and perplexing cancer.

Only here in this basement with his parakeet will we figure this one out.

There is a blood test for recurrent carcinoid tumor, and his astute specialist had done this test, the chromogranin A level. But as so often happens, the level was equivocal, slightly elevated but not clearly high. The test added nothing to the clinical guessing we were already doing. The CT scan of the abdomen did not show a tumor, but carcinoid can be tiny, just 1cm, and still metastasize and secrete hormones, so it does not always show up on radiographs either. We would need to spend time with Tom at home, discovering when the symptoms came on, building trust so he would share if he were finding narcotics surreptitiously.

I work with a health coach. She calls and visits the less sick patients during the times when I am not there. She can spend even more time in the home, building trust, and listening. My team's coach, Lara, is a middle-aged woman who has a grown disabled son not too dissimilar from Tom. She has the wisdom of the ancients, born of her life that did not turn out as planned, but did turn out somehow. Lara does not label him, or fire him when he has an angry outburst. Tom learns to call when he has an "attack" and we do a lot of IV bags of fluid in his basement, and he avoids the hospital across the street, and the system saves thousands and thousands of dollars. And we may even solve his medical mystery here too.

Does it take the empathy developed by suffering yourself through a similar illness to actually connect with complex patients? I know I would not be here if I did not have my own complex patient at home, my son, whom I have learned from and who has formed all the wisdom that I contain. I suppose I was destined for this type of medicine when my son became ill and disabled. I learned about dedication, which our current medical system does not encourage. It's not impossible to find the dedicated in clinics and hospitals, but the dedicated soon become discouraged by the pressures of time and billing. Dedication takes time; it is defined by time.

Living in the Numbers

"We can't possibly know (let alone keep track of) the tremendous number of mechanical influences on our behavior because we inhabit an extraordinarily complicated machine." -- Daniel Wegner, The Illusion of Conscious Will

Out on the eastern edge of Portland, before it turns into Gresham via some bureaucratic sleight-of-hand, there are streets without sidewalks, and a house where a man works on a car. The car is pulled up along the side of the road, the socket set and other tools are strewn around it, not in wheeled chests, but in the dirt. There is a sign, hand lettered, reading "car repair". The man is missing nearly all his teeth except the front two. He greets me with a smile showing teeth and gums. He is the grandson of Ms N, who is my patient and has had a cough for the past week.

For many people a cough is a minor annoyance. But when you have full kidney failure and are dependent on dialysis to filter your blood daily, when you have diabetes that caused the kidney failure in the first place, when you have a heart that squeezes only at half its normal capacity, then a cough can be the prelude to catastrophe. By intervening early in the course of destabilization, we can sometimes prevent the dangerous instabilities that lead to hospitalizations and ICU stays.

I am led into the house. The door opens to the living room. The house is dirty. In fact, the house appears to be made of dirt. How can there be smeared muddy footprints up the wall past the doorknob? There is a couch. It is a low couch, and perhaps does not have legs. It is covered with soiled garments and bits of cloth. The room is dark and the linens are darker, and I cannot tell if they are clothes, or sheets, or automotive rags. In the back room I hear squabbling children. This place is on the edge. The edge of what, I am not sure.

"Here's my grandma, she's back in her bedroom. I called yesterday because I am worried about her cough." The grandson leads me to the right, into a bedroom, and then disappears back outside to attend to the car.

Dirt, squalor and poverty immediately conjure their presumed consequences: carelessness, broken families and violence. Except here it is backwards. The toothless grandson, haplessly trying to make ends meet by fixing wrecks parked in mud puddles, cares for this grandma, and called for help, appropriately.

She emerges from a pile of blankets, pale, grey, skin like the winter Portland sky. Renal failure and dialysis always create this complexion; she is not necessarily decompensating and acutely ill. The kidneys secrete hormones that cause blood cell production in the bones, so without functioning kidneys, everyone becomes mildly anemic and pale. Then, the dialysis filter is not quite as good as the healthy kidney, so the toxin level is always higher in the body. And dialysis patients never have energy, so they do not go outside, rarely sit in the sun, and never exercise. They become ghosts of their former selves, grey and wraithlike. Those who choose to fight because they have something to live for can survive for years like this. Others say "enough" and stop dialysis, slipping within weeks into a peaceful coma and completing their transition to another world.

Ms N is fighting it, and has for the past year since she started peritoneal dialysis. There are two ways to artificially filter blood without kidneys, hemodialysis - hooking a vein to a machine which pumps blood through a filter, and peritoneal, where a permanent plastic tube is sewn through the abdominal wall into the empty cavity around the intestines. Salt water is dripped into the normally empty spaces every night, and then drained out in the mornings. While the fluid sits in the peritoneal cavity, the surrounding blood vessels automatically exchange out their toxins and they get drained away. This method is much simpler and uses the body's own tissues as the filter. It can be done at home, but has to be done every night as it is not as efficient as the blood filtering type which normally only requires 3 runs per week. Ms N does peritoneal dialysis at home, and her grandson religiously records her blood pressure, temperature and weight in a neat notebook every morning, required by the medical equipment provider. The toothless grandson with the scattered tools has done a better job with the dialysis machine than most medical assistants I work with.

"Ms N, I am Dr. Benson, so nice to meet you!" I start with a greeting and a handshake.

"What are you doing here?" she asks as she extracts a pale hand from the sheets.

"Your grandson called yesterday because he was worried about your cough," I explain as I realize she was not expecting me. "Are you doing ok?" Her grandson did not tell her he had called. Grandma has a room in the house; she is kept alive only by the dint of will of the family, religiously changing bags of fluids every night and recording arcane numbers. And yet, the muddled communications of caring appear more like the mud puddles outside.

“I’ve been coughing,” she begins and we settle into the routine of doctor and patient, a universal back and forth, honed by thousands of years of tradition. She is used to doctors stopping by because someone from my team does so at least monthly. Ms N has uncontrolled diabetes, vascular disease in her legs, kidney failure and heart disease. She has practically lived at some of the local hospitals. On any given day, if she shows up in an emergency room, her laboratory tests will be wildly abnormal, her skin looks “sick” and she likely will have some complaints. She will always get admitted due to worries about something, and she will stay for at least a week while the hospital team tries in vain to “improve” her various diseases. So we visit frequently and keep her away from the emergency room.

Diabetes destroys kidneys, and Ms N routinely used to have blood sugars in the 4-500 range. She ate her traditional diet that became constricted since she moved to this area without a real grocery store nearby -- a so-called “food desert”. Urban planning creates an ever denser downtown for Portland. Wealth and jobs create rising cost of living in the central, desirable regions close to restaurants, coffee shops and like-minded tech workers. The immigrants, the poor, and the minorities who once lived there now live farther and farther east, out where the sidewalks end. Eighty-second avenue used to demarcate the eastern edge of urban Portland. Now, there is no edge as the higher-numbered streets blend into the sprawling suburbs of Gresham and Boring. People here are said to live "In the Numbers"; that is, in the numbers higher than about 122nd Ave. Today I am out in the numbers.

After years of uncontrolled diabetes, the kidneys frequently fail. Dialysis is now initiated in 90,000 people per year in America. It is outrageously cost-intensive, and yet paid for by Medicare, out of public funds. Without dialysis, Ms N would die. Disease seems to exist on a spectrum of personal responsibility. At one end are childhood cancers, such as leukemia, that seem to strike randomly and tragically, and no one would possibly "blame" the kid seen in the fund-raising advertisements, bald and slender, trailing an oxygen tube. On the other end of the spectrum appear diseases where we blame the sufferers: alcoholism, and morbid obesity. I have never seen an ad attempting to elicit sympathy and collect funds for an obesity clinic.

As science catches up with our popular conceptions, the spectrum of responsibility becomes muddled. We realize that all disease has a genetic component, even these ones where we ask, "How could he have done that to himself?" Over the next few decades we will certainly learn more about the complex cascade of genes that cause some people to suffer while others escape with exactly the same behaviors. Doctors continually tread the fine line between cajoling patients into changing their lifestyles and attempting to avoid blaming people for their diseases. Society and politics also attempt to parse this grey zone by alternatingly imposing penalties for using the social safety net or ranting about structural inequalities, depending on the party in power.

Outside the bedroom the kids are running around and yelling. "I wish they would not make so much noise," Ms N proclaims wearily. "Sharma does not live here anyway, but she makes the most racket. She lives out back in the trailer, but her old man ain't around much."

We examine her dialysis catheter site. It is a clean hole, right into the abdomen, with a clear plastic tube that disappears into the nether world of internal organs. Not infected. A black hole from the comprehensible world of kids, blankets and grandsons, into the universe of doctors, pill bottles and notebooks full of daily blood pressures. It's the pipe that connects my world to this patient's world. Without the dialysis catheter I would not be here, invited into this home on the edge, sharing a moment of poverty and hope that feels raw to me. Diabetes leads to kidney failure leads to a surgeon poking a hole through the wall between an Oregon redneck and her doctor.

I check all the carefully written numbers in her vitals notebook. The dialysis company will stop providing her fluids and take back the machine if the records are not kept properly. And they are proper, in neat rows, without a smudge. It is the only clean place in the house, this notebook and these pages. I peer out the grimy window to the front and there is the grandson, his head under the upraised hood, leaning in.

I listen with the stethoscope to the bases of the lungs. They are decreased, with a few fine crackles. Most people on dialysis end up with some extra fluid that makes its way into crevices and crannies around the body. The crackles likely represent small "pleural effusions", or some of the extra fluid in a small pocket around the base of the lungs. Almost certainly this is what was causing the slight cough, as the fluid irritates the lung lining and triggers the cough reflex.

She could have taken better care of her diabetes. Or, better yet, eaten better and exercised more and never had diabetes. "I used to live down in southwest Portland, but my grandson moved me up here." I wonder what her neighborhood was like down there and if there were grocery stores. Out here they seem to close as fast as new pharmacies seem to open. Perhaps Americans buy more medicines than food these days, and these all-night pharmacies stock all the essentials anyways: canned hotdogs, chips and 3 aisles of soda. We could all do better with the cards that we are dealt, yet some people are dealt a very poor hand indeed.

"Thanks for calling me and letting me come in," I manage to say as I collect my gear. It sounds odd, and it is not something I usually say as I am leaving a patient's house. But I have received my blessing, and it is now time to leave.

Becoming the Medicine Man

"Ts'its'tsi'nako, Thought-Woman, is sitting in her room and whatever she thinks about diappears... 'I will tell you something about stories, They aren't just entertainment. Don't be fooled. They are all we have, you see, all we have to fight off illness and death.'" -- *Leslie Marmon Silko, Ceremony*

There are a row of trailer parks along Halsey Boulevard as Gresham becomes Fairview becomes Troutdale out on the eastern fringes of the city. The trailers are old, with small patches of grass and populated with pickup trucks. Just to the north runs the main railroad line out of Portland and up the gorge, to Eastern Oregon and the rest of America. Every few hours 10,000 tons of steel and paper towel rolls barrel through, their presence felt not by a whistle, but by a long low vibration of the earth. This is the artery where America mainlines Chinese imports, injected directly into the heartland from the Port of Portland. Near the tracks, these ramshackle rusting buildings were once meant to be cheap temporary developments on the edge of the industrial parks. And like everything temporary in the American West, they have come to define the landscape.

Diego lives here with his wife. They have a small blue trailer with cluttered steps, a cluttered yard and a cluttered interior.

"¡Buenas tardes doctor!" he greets me with enthusiasm. "¿Cómo ha estado?"

"Bien, y ¿Usted?" We exchange pleasantries and reconnect at his kitchen table. He is a large man, and has gotten larger since retiring from construction ten years ago. He used to lay subfloors with a certain specialized type of epoxy, as much as I can gather. Now his wife works at the McDonalds down the road, and he mostly sits at home. He immigrated from Jalisco, Mexico as a young man, pursuing work. And he found it, on his knees day after day, building the American dream for years. His English is very poor and it's difficult for him to negotiate the various doctor's instructions from his many appointments.

"Ya no salgo mucho," he admits. He has diabetes, and a limited understanding of how his traditional diet, which served him well as a laborer, plates of tortillas with tamales, soda on the hot days, is now slowly imprisoning him in a cage of obesity and a row of pill bottles. To qualify for this program of home visits, a patient must have at least five chronic conditions, and Diego has seven. So even with an hour visit, we cannot talk about everything. We focus on the diabetes and his blood sugars. He is dedicated to compliance and organizes his medications on a shelf by the table. He checks his sugars three times daily. In the morning when he awakens, the numbers are good, about 100. But by late afternoon they are up to 250 to 300. This means his body is appropriately compensated overnight when there is no new sugar coming in, no food eaten. But throughout the day, his pancreas cannot keep up with the carbohydrates that he consumes. His obese body is "insulin resistant"so his blood sugar level slowly creeps up. The high blood levels of sugars then cause chemical reactions with the glucose attaching itself to nerves numbing the feeling in his feet, and attracting cholesterol to the walls of arteries, causing the heart attack he had last year.

I imagine the medicine man reconnects a human to their place, their community and culture, thereby making someone whole again. I wish I were a medicine man, reconnecting this man to something. Instead I am a physician, visiting homes to provide medical care. Not to everyone's homes, just to the most frail and elderly.

It is too expensive to send doctors to everyone's homes, so we find only the most complex patients, the ones who constantly cycle through hospitals and emergency rooms, the ones who have a page-long list of medications, and a book full of subspecialists all vying for supremacy of their particular organ. These most frail and complex patients rarely benefit from more care; they have been overly medicalized already, losing some humanity along the way. So I attempt to provide holistic care, meeting the patient as a person, in their house. Meeting the patient in their literal home so as to find their spiritual home. Currently, 10% of patients consume 50% of our health care dollars. We simply spend more on these people whose physical health is related to their mental health, and their environment, and their opportunities, and…, and… Routine care works well for most people, but we now have a subset of Americans who are "super-utilizers", who have so many complex conditions that the ten minute office visit with primary care or specialist simply adds to their complexity rather than solving any of their problems. These are my patients, and I love them.

People who are sick often become lost under the fluorescent lights of a sterile medical system. So my job is to reconnect to a person, who lives in a place. Is from a place. I think that is what it means to be a soul. Souls don't flit around the gauzy ether like cherubim in Renaissance paintings. They appear very solid to me, and actually more rooted to their places, like trees which grow in the right climate. I do not suppose that the medicine man "cures" old people from dying any more than I do. Death will come for us all. The diabetes and the blocked arteries would not disappear through spiritual connection, but those illnesses would not define the individual. They would simply become an aspect of their life.

Down the hill from this place lies Blue Lake, and on its west shore "Kwakiutl" where a placard states that a Native village used to exist. The spot is wondrously situated, a wise choice for siting a village. Mt Hood shouts from the distance across the still waters, just to the north lies the Columbia, and although most of this area can be swampy lowlands in the rainy season, here there are rocky outcroppings that allow a pleasant airy breeze. Lewis and Clark apparently paddled down the Columbia past this very spot. We find in their journals the first mention of this village. Except that it had already been destroyed by a smallpox epidemic, expedition's arrival. Waves of smallpox raced ahead of the European contact, waves of death from every interaction.

Looking across the lake with ripples gently caressing the pink lilies, I cannot imagine the horror of your entire village dying in front of you. Out of nowhere, your son gets a headache, then fever and bleeding, skin sores. The disease progresses rapidly with delirium: the brain moving into a different world before the body dies and follows it. The medicine man must have tried everything that he knew: dances, masks, ceremonies. Apparently nothing worked and a whole people died. A whole people. Why was this disease so deadly? We make sense of it all now by inventing theories like a "lack of innate immunity." We like to make sense of complexity for it otherwise leaves an unsettled sensation in the heart.

Visitors to Blue Lake occasionally discover, by wandering on a small out-of-the-way path, that this place has a history beyond barbecues and church picnics. Blue Lake Park, situated out "in the numbers", far from the gentrification of downtown Portland, has become the immigrant park. Here, there are vast picnic areas where Saudis and Ukrainians and Vietnamese come for community picnics. The immigrant communities of eastern Portland find a temporary home here on the weekends, where they gather and prepare food from all over the world. The park has welcomed this role by placing signage in Russian and Vietnamese. On weekdays I have met babushkas here, fishing at the lakeside, who eagerly smile and point to what they have caught as I walk by, a gathering spot for grandmas to spend the day, and perhaps to bring home dinner for the clan. How fitting that this spot where the first immigrants paddled past is now the immigrant park. How fitting that the park connects immigrant communities to the larger community and the land that sometimes seems hostile. How utterly tragic that it all began in destruction.

Back up the hill from the long lost Kwakiutl village, Diego and I discuss blood sugars and the foods that cause it to rise. Most people do not realize that insulin is a natural hormone whose main purpose is to create fat cells. Insulin facilitates the passage of sugar from the bloodstream into cells where it is converted into lipids -- fat. So we can control blood sugars with extra insulin injections, but the consequences will be an expanding waistline. For most diabetics, the solution is not more insulin, but less food and more exercise, which is an "insulin-free" means of burning blood sugar. This trailer park is hemmed in by train tracks and a freeway. There are no sidewalks. Diego has a bad knee and it hurts him to walk much anyway. His exercise consists of trips from the bedroom, through the kitchen to the living room and the television. His ten foot yard is full of all the stuff that won't fit in the trailer. This place is killing him.

Time Becomes Meaningless in the Face of Creativity

"Traditional cultures used to value their outlying personalities, listen to them carefully, and believe they had a direct line of communication to the spirit world. We not only don't listen to them, we rush to the pill cabinet to shut them up as quickly as possible." -- Anonymous online comment from an Autism forum

Ms. C lives in subsidized housing in the crowded northwest district of downtown. Outside of the upscale Pearl, but down below the truly upscale places that rise up onto the west hills. She is bipolar, or has bipolar disease, in the more respectful formulation. Doctors equate diseases with people as a form of shorthand in order to keep track of a busy practice. The metonymy of "The head trauma in room 3", and the "diabetic in the waiting room" are not so damaging or insulting to patients as they are destructive to ourselves as they nibble away at our humanity. I would say that

Ms. C suffers from bipolar disease, except that most of the time she enjoys it.

She sits in her small living room like a spider in the center of her web. Stretching out from her chair are lines of oxygen tubing to various scattered tanks and concentrating apparatuses. Some of them might even work. There is a small end table with watercolor paints and paper dripping off the edges onto the floor. The walls to her left are bookshelves from floor to ceiling. "I used to teach English, everything 19th century was my specialty." Confabulation goes with the territory of bipolar, but the titles seem to bear witness to a career of struggling with long convoluted novels: Dickens, Proust, Joyce. I do not associate the up-all-night mania with crashing through long texts, but why not? Prose that might put most of us to sleep would hardly be noticed in the midst of full delirium.

She wears the uniform of the housebound -- sweatpants and sweatshirt, baggy, comfortable, entirely unconcerned with the world's gaze. We exchange pleasantries and then launch straight in to checking on the medications that she is supposed to be taking. There are a few different lists, from different doctors, at different times: the hospital from last year, the urgent care she visited while traveling out to Michigan to see her sister who had leukemia, the primary care office, the handwritten in pencil list of medications that she had gathered from research on Google... The line between wishful and real blurs in the rush of thought and speech.

"I just don't have the energy I used to," she complains. "I had to start this oxygen last year. I really don't like it, you know? It's confining. My pills got really messed up when I went out to Michigan. The pharmacy here was doing a pill-pack, but then I needed refills out there, so some are in the pill-pack, but some are just bottles, and they won't refill those until February 12th, that's what they said."

There are medicine bottles in a small toiletries bag. One of those is empty and lists "oxybutynin", a bladder medication which is featured on none of the lists. She laughs, "Now I was putting the clopidogrel in there, don't worry, that is not what it says on it, but I needed a place to put the extra pills after I got back, and I didn't have a place in the bag..." She continues, but the explanation clarifies nothing. I am worried. There are a few pills packaged in wonderful little baggies, attached together in a roll by the pharmacy, labelled and dated for "Friday 8am" and "Friday noon" and so forth. Looking just at this small box with its elegant labelled roll, the world appears coherent again, just for a minute.

To the right are two walls covered with haphazardly placed artwork. Some have frames, some are just taped to the wall. The colors are bright, vivid greens and reds in large areas. They brighten the room, and my interest brightens Ms. C's face. "My niece painted that at 8 years old! Here she is now, she is twelve," and she points to a framed photo in another area. "Would you like some tea?"

Bipolar disease, or manic-depression, is common. There are two forms, type 1 and type 2. In type 1, people become completely manic to the level of psychosis, with endless run-on speech, inability to sleep, and usually socially outrageous actions such as stealing cars, sleeping with 10 people in one night and so on. I always ask, "Have you ever been arrested?" And if the answer is yes, then they probably have type 1. Type 2 is defined by "hypomania", or mildly elevated levels of activity and pressured speech, but maintaining basic social functioning. Ms. C clearly has type 2, and has managed to translate her disability into a remarkable life. Many do not do as well, and struggle to maintain happiness.

"I never needed oxygen until this year," she begins. "I want to do more. Sometimes I am just stuck here." I am having difficulty sorting out which medications she takes and which she does not. Some on her list will really help her heart failure and breathing, not to mention her mania and episodes of severe depression.

"So... let's start again with the trip to Michigan. Here is the candesartan bottle; is this the one you ran out of at that time?" I ask.

"Oh yes, that is the one. Can you believe my poor sister, she got leukemia and the chemo treatments were so hard, I just had to go out there. The weather was miserable, you think we have it bad here in Portland, you can't imagine Michigan. I used to teach out there, you know. I really liked those classes, that college just let me do what I wanted. My favorite was a class called 'composition' and those kids didn't complain when we read poetry..."

I interrupted, "Let's get back to the medicine again, I want to put all the medicines that are not packaged already by the pharmacy into this pile here, and the others we are going to put in the little blue bag. Let's put these away. Tomorrow I am going to have our pharmacist help you get back to having all the pills put in the PillPack by the pharmacy."

We went back and forth a few times. Our team has a pharmacist who does home visits as well. We also have social workers and dieticians and nurses. It takes a village sometimes to keep people at home. It feels good to be a part of a village that helps people live at home, at the center of their own spider webs.

How would her life have unfolded without bipolar disease? Is that a question that is even worth asking? Is that like asking what would have happened if I had turned left at that light instead of right? Or is it more like asking, what would I be like if I had not had a disabled son? This is a remarkable woman, who would have perhaps accomplished more on a certain level without her bipolar, yet does not see herself as held back by it. "This getting old is really hard," she said, "but I am actually really enjoying it." And she smiled. Just a little manic is a great place to be.

Knickknacks in Gresham

"Where are your stomping grounds?" --sign on the wall of a Troutdale coffee house

"Come in, come in!" says the old grandma as she opens the door into her immaculate house. She is small. And active. Grandma Ethel buzzes around her house, back and forth, sitting then standing at the table while I put down my bag and open my laptop to start our visit. "Let me make you some coffee..."

One might suppose that such a vigorous active person would not qualify for home-based medical care. And certainly many patients are disabled enough not to be able to get out to doctors, but that is not the main reason to do home visits. The home is where health is created, or destroyed. Looking back at the years I spent trying to do healthcare in clinics and hospital rooms, I marvel that I did not give up earlier. In health care facilities everything is set up for the convenience of the system. There is a waiting room, a check-in, a schedule, a series of small sterile rooms closely packed to allow quick turn-around. Everything extraneous has been removed that does not contribute to the efficiency with which human bodies are shuttled through the health assembly line. In these systems, the human is reduced entirely to a body. Only the body, and perhaps a few scraps of clothes in clinics, and not even those in the hospital, enters the sterile innards of the health establishment. Only the body is treated and then only the body exits out the other end after it is tapped, prodded, measured, cut, stuck and stamped.

Sitting at Grandma Ethel's table, the power relationship was reversed. She was in charge, serving me coffee, standing by my side while I laboriously booted up my computer system and accessed her chart, clucking and tsk, tsking as it all took so long. The woman and her house were clearly inseparable. Every wall, which was of course papered with a stripes and paisley pattern not seen anywhere since 1972, was covered with shelves, and the shelves were covered with figurines, and the figurines were porcelain animals and children cavorting colorfully in energetic poses. My practical gaze wandered the spotless the shelves. The dusting alone would be intimidating, to lift each figurine, to carefully dust it and under it, to place it back, just so. From my seat at the table I made out two other rooms, identically shellacked with knickknacks and brown shag carpet. I had entered a slow-motion bee hive: immobile and timeless in its ceramic stillness, yet requiring near constant energy and motion to maintain.

My coffee was poured, so I had to begin. “How are you today, Mrs. Ethel?”

“Oh what am I going to do about Jeanie? She is in high school this year, and I am so worried.”

Some people answer my opening question with their aches and pains. Others respond, like this, not talking about themselves at all. Jeanie is the grand-daughter, and lives here because her mother is a meth addict who Ethel kicked out many years ago. Ethel’s “body” that I was sent here to treat was not confined to her small wiry physical form. It extends to the house with the white picket fence, the figurines, the old carpet, and the bedroom in the back where a teenage girl is maturing and trying to make sense of her absent mother and time-warped grandma.

Ethel had high blood pressure and a lot of anxiety. Most people with elevated blood pressure end up needing multiple medications for adequate control. And despite seeming to be a simple physiologic process, understanding what controls blood pressure, and why it is important for health, has remained stubbornly difficult for medical science. Blood exits from the heart into the aorta, the large artery an inch or two in diameter that arches up from the heart and then down along the chest, through the abdomen and finally divides into two arteries coursing down each leg. Along the way, numerous smaller branches emerge at right angles, usually one for each major organ: stomach, small intestines, kidneys, large intestines, etc. However, it is not this system of larger hoses that controls the pressure, instead it is the much smaller, microscopic arterioles that collectively, in their millions, dilate or contract to control the flow of blood and its pressure. Paradoxically, the risk from high blood pressure in the smaller arterioles damages the larger arteries, thickening their walls, causing cholesterol plaque to build up and rupture, causing heart attacks and strokes.

Methamphetamines have been synthesized by humans since the late 1800's, and exert their effects by displacing our normal neurotransmitter hormones from nerve endings, causing them to release at inappropriate times. The effect is one of a huge burst of "fight-or-flight" hormones into the entire body: that rush of adrenaline, accompanied by energy, euphoria, often careening over into hallucinations, and paranoia.

In a terrible irony, the meth caused Ethel's daughter to share her mother's diagnosis for hypertension, just from entirely different causes. Meth creates an adrenaline surge that constricts the vessels, which is part of the reason why meth can permanently damage the heart, requiring it to pump against a huge pressure load, thickening it and wearing it out.

"My daughter started doing meth in high school I think," Ethel explained. "I didn't know she was doing it. She didn't tell me anything! Sometimes she acted strangely, but she was a teenager, you know"

"Have you lived here since then?" I ask.

"Oh yes, we have lived in this house since 1969. My husband got a job out here doing transportation. And we have stayed." She is quiet for a moment, reflecting, then adds, "She looked tired a lot back then." She wrings her hands and fidgets, her body reflecting the agitation of her powerlessness in the face of impending doom.

"Right away she got pregnant. Jeanie was born, but that didn't stop her, she kept getting high."

Meth can be ingested into the body through nearly every orifice and in every way: eaten, smoked, snorted, injected or stuffed into the vagina. The thinner the membrane or skin between the drug and the blood stream, the faster it is absorbed and its effects felt. Unlike heroin, which quickly creates increased receptors and physiological dependency, thus rendering the user instantly an "addict", meth can smolder along, with less than daily use. And because the user is not quite so intimately constrained by daily use, spinning their lives completely out of control, the meth user can keep going for years, or decades. We have geriatric meth use now, with toothless old men in their 70's still showing up using, looking for one more chance to feel "forever young."

The chaos of methamphetamines seems entirely incongruous to the excessive orderliness of this home and these over-dusted shelves. Did the tidy housekeeping evolve to ward off the internal struggle of watching a life fall apart, or did the daughter's rebellion against structure manifest in the destruction of meth? Doctors like to imagine that we deal in a science of cause and effect, that we are elucidating the causes of pathological processes in our patients so that we can reverse them and effect a cure. It is mostly an illusion.

Medical science, starting from its origins in a laboratory with pathways of protein interactions, and leading to large-scale randomized trials, is able to ferret out physiological routes that are clearly causal. But out here on the boulevard, where the potential variables affecting health multiply exponentially, the best we can do is use the known causal pathways as ships might use lighthouses guarding distant but dangerous rocks. They mark a few known points in a mostly dangerous and unknown sea. Medical science continually commits the error of overstating its gains in knowledge by equating them with scientific advances. With every physiologic pathway we map out, from the oncogene in colon cancer to the fully sequenced human genome, we trumpet our apparent control over human health. And time after time, the reality out on the boulevard is that bodies and minds turn out to be more complex, that one more brilliant pathway is just that, one more point of light in a vast complex sea.

Ethel took care of Jeanie right from her birth. The daughter was able to stay away from meth and her meth crowd for a few weeks at the most. So Ethel, at age 50, started over as a mother, raising her granddaughter, as so many grandmothers have.

“Kicking her out of here was the hardest thing I ever did,” she muses, still standing beside the kitchen table. “It was the best thing to do. Jeanie deserves a chance too. And now she is a sophomore. And I am an old woman, what do I know of her concerns? She is always on that phone... Are those kids doing meth, and sleeping around? A lot of those kids are just hanging around up there at the mall, I don’t know what they are doing.”

I work at the computer and we plan which medication to adjust because some physiological pathway claims it will dilate Ethel’s arterioles a little more and bring down her blood pressure. I will try not to make the error of treating this blood pressure as just a bunch of chemical pathways.

The Sun Mask

"A man lived at Yê'kwin. He said that he had come down from above, being the son of the Sun. He had the name SE'nlê?. Then he wore the sun mask. He came after he had left the place from which he came down, where he had first been. He searched for a house site, looking for a good country. Then he found Bar-at-Mouth-of-River. There he built a house on the meadow back of the point of Bar-at-Mouth-of-River. Then he took off his sun mask and he became an ordinary man there."
--Traditional Pacific Coast story collected in 1893 by Franz Boas

Layer after layer I unwrap the bandages from the lower leg. The dry outer gauze hides the inner saturated layer, gummy and curdled. The odor escapes before being released by the last turning: a sickly sweet cloying dagger that cuts into the nose and lungs and brings bile to the throat. The smell clings to clothes and to one's memory. Once experienced, never forgotten. *Pseudomonas aeruginosa* is a virulent bacterium that putrefies flesh and emits the odor of death. Everyone in healthcare knows this smell, and we know it from across the room, down the hall, and back in our memories to that first time when as quivering students, we were exposed to the brutal reality of pure sickness that textbooks only conjure up in small hints.

I am unwrapping the dressing from a diabetic foot wound. Diabetes, with its unregulated molecules of glucose swarming the bloodstream, destroys nerves in the feet, and decreases circulation, and short-circuits infection-fighting white cells. The result is insensate feet that are easily injured by a bump or bruise or simply a slip of a toenail scissor. The wound does not heal, the millions of colonizing skin bacteria sense their chance and invade the deeper moist tissues, setting up shop and multiplying until the wound deepens and becomes a crater. For the unlucky, the bacteria that predominate will be *Pseudomonas*. The penetrating smell would drive most people from their home, so some simply wrap it up and ignore it.

Every time I encounter this particular experience, the face-to-face confrontation with decay, it feels like the first time again, so long ago now. I was a medical student, on the road to fulfilling my desire to emulate Albert Schweitzer. I had matched at a residency based in a community health center in Colorado. The diabetic foot, with its thinning skin, and built up callouses, and painless broken bones, and endless infections, became my teacher.

Community health centers are remarkable institutions that provide medical care on a sliding scale fee schedule in medically underserved areas. Most doctors flock to wealthy regions, and cultural hubs. Poor rural and inner-city areas cannot compete, so they set up these grant funded institutions to provide some care to people who otherwise would have none. The most dedicated nurses, doctors and social workers come to these places to ply their craft. They are the plaster that attempts to plug the ever-widening cracks in the American health care system. The community health center is strangely analogous to the diabetic foot: an unforeseen consequence existing on the periphery of a dysregulated larger system.

The community health center, or Federally Qualified Health Center (FQHC) in the lingo, is an amazing institution that few appreciate for its role in raising our healthcare out of what would otherwise be an entirely third world, banana republic, system. The wealthy will always buy access to health services, both here and in the poorest country in the world. The poor cannot afford the market price for healthcare so end up suffering in the gutter. The FQHC saves lives, lowers costs and functions as a true safety net in our society. However, it still functions in an antiquated manner. The centers are paid by the volume of people they see -- even though a part of these funds come from grants -- and then the providers are paid in the same way. In order to be solvent, you have to see more people, and then bill more. Like any economic game, there is a minimum volume required in order to pay the expenses. The overhead is high, so to stay in the black, providers have to see 20 patients per day, or more. My FQHC provided excellent training because I saw many really sick patients, endlessly, back to back. It was crazy.

I underwent the scourge of residency, with its long nights and scientific discipline. I then served in the National Health Service Corps in rural Wyoming, honing my skills in a harsh environment, without all the tertiary care backup that most take for granted. Later, I spent most of my career in a hospital, caring for people in snapshots of 3-4 days while they were admitted for acute illnesses. I patched them up, discharged them, washed my hands literally and metaphorically, and moved on. And then saw how they just came back a few weeks later, with the same problems, or other ones. A master of human physiology, I was rarely solving actual human issues. So I jumped at the chance to do home visits in an environment where we focus on savings rather than the fee-for-service billings of normal medical care. Insurance companies need our services because only a few very complex, high-cost patients, account for as much as 40% of the expenses of an entire cohort of people. So we get to do whatever is necessary for patients without worrying about billing, usually by keeping them at home, and focusing on their goals rather than the medical establishment's "health" goals.

Every time I smell *Pseudomonas*, I recall my entire process of medical training and the route that brought me here to Portland, to my own Bar-at-Mouth-of-River. I cling to an apocryphal piece of family lore that my father's grandmother's mother was descended from a Native tribe in Quebec. Ultimately it would not really matter even if it were true, as heritage is more about culture and less about genetics. The ancestors that I am certain of are Norwegian and Swedish. And my medical clogs, the ones I used to wear around the hospital, the ones everyone wears around every hospital in the world, are made in Denmark. My blue eyes define me as more related to Lewis and Clark than to the Kwakiutl before them or the Vietnamese of today. Am I a medicine man? Perhaps our imagined Native heritage can help to save our current broken medical system, and rootless culture and lost people. We need some blazes on the trail to lead us out of our rootlessness towards a more authentic way of being human.

I am sitting with another infected diabetic foot, and with the person connected to that foot. Trying to stay connected to it. If we cannot control the infection because the arterial blood supply is already too clogged, or the bacteria too resistant after multiple rounds of antibiotics, then amputating the foot will be the only means to prevent infection from spreading into the bloodstream and killing the entire body. I put on my Sun Mask and offer words of encouragement.

"Here is the plan: we will peel off the infected layers of the wound right now, then I will have the home health nurse come out here every day to change the bandages. We will start the right antibiotics today. I have looked at your medicine list and the one I am starting will be safe with the other things you are taking. Now, the blood pressure in your legs that I measured today is less than the blood pressure in your arms, so we need to be sure your circulation is ok, and I am going to have you see the vascular surgeon to be certain we can't do a procedure to improve the blood flow. And you need to have excellent blood sugar control so your white cells can fight the infection properly.

"That is a lot of stuff, I know. But don't worry, we are going to be with you through this entire thing. Tomorrow the wound-care nurse will be here. My case manager nurse will be calling and asking you about your blood sugars and helping to schedule your vascular surgery appointment."

After I leave the house I take off my Sun Mask by putting away my stethoscope. I become once again an ordinary man, returning to my own house at the confluence of the Willamette and Columbia rivers, my Bar-at-Mouth-of-River. I have my own complex chronic son Noah at home who has inspired me to try to be a good doctor more than any so-called role model that I may have read about or met. I may succeed with this Pseudomonas and save this foot connected to a body, but I have not succeeded with Noah, and that leaves an internal raw space for me. I wear the Sun Mask to hide the tears from Noah not getting to grow up and run around like other kids, not getting to talk and babble about pipes and machines like he did before the seizures hit. The Sun Mask has served me well and I think it has served the thousands of patients I have seen, and the few that I have actually helped. Native stories always seem to contain the character of the trickster, sometimes Raven, or Coyote or some other sly animal. I am beginning to understand these legends now. Every day I trick my patients into believing I am the Sun God who controls destinies and can heal their woes. And every day I trick myself into believing the same thing. And every day my family tricks itself into thinking that Noah will get better, and his seizures will stop and his motor control will improve and he will jump up and run around with his brother like he did as an infant. Life without the trickster would be a poor impoverished journey indeed. We need the trickster so very much.

I would like to understand how I came to be wearing this Sun Mask, how despite no training, no skill, despite centuries of willful misunderstanding, I came to be working as an imitation medicine man in Portland. My patients see me with my “sun mask” still on, but I am an ordinary man who settled down here at the mouth of the river, amongst the moss and April blossoms and grey January half-light, searching for a good country, like everyone else.

Between Popeyes and Martin Luther King

"The notion that writing about race, which is to say, the force of white supremacy, is marginal and provincial is itself parcel to white supremacy, premised on the notion that the foundational crimes of this country are mostly irrelevant to its existence."
--Ta-Nehesi Coates, We Were Eight Years in Power

No one answers our knock, so we wait on the porch with its peeling blue railing. Northeast Portland along Martin Luther King Jr Avenue is resplendent on a sunny September afternoon. The bright boulevard with patchy dried flower beds awaits its annual winter soaking in a secure dormancy. October and its rains have never, ever failed in Portland. Now, the western sun strikes the house and creates shade on the porch as we wait for Mrs. J.

Standing on the porch, we wonder what to do. She confirmed yesterday by phone that she knew about our appointment today here at her house. We call again. This time, she answers her cell phone. She is on the bus, returning from her few daily hours as a caregiver to some other elderly person. She has eight chronic conditions, with Parkinson's disease, and her fingers shake as she talks, yet she herself finds meaning, and a few dollars, in a job caring for others.

When she arrives, we find we are all locked out. Unperturbed by her inability to enter her own house, we talk on the porch where she sits on a rickety chair and we lean on the railing. With Parkinsons, everything slows down. Her movements are slow, her speech is slow. I can't understand half of what she says and lean close. She speaks at half speed, with the rounded mellow African-American accent. It is an accent that is more difficult, and more foreign, to me than Mexican and Cuban. Such is our post-modern predicament that I feel more at home on another continent than a few blocks away just off Martin Luther King Jr Avenue. Thus is Portland famous, or infamous, for being "America's whitest city".

She has trouble remembering her medication list, and has been fired from her primary care provider because she does not keep track of appointments and has missed too many. She mistrusts the medical world and was told that Parkinson's medications were "poisoning her." So her hands shake, and she complains of dropping her money. She had paid her bus fare, but forgot to put the other bills in her purse. As her Parkinson hands shook, her money fell, and she arrived home without it.

“My nephew was getting some chicken,” she said. “We goin’ to have a real nice dinner.”

“Hey white boy! I see you there.” We hear an angry voice from around the side of the house. A disheveled man appears, talking to himself and occasionally calling out to us. He is angry, angry to see us lounging on the porch.

“Oh that’s my brother,” Mrs. J says, “don’t pay him no mind, he always do that.”

“Is he alright?” I nervously ask, as he waves his arms around, really asking, am I alright and safe here?

“He’s not right in the head. He’s ok.”

He wandered off, cursing at me. She explains that her brother has schizophrenia, and lives with her in this house, along with five other people variously related to her. So she is correct; her brother is both not right in the head, and ok.

After all, what am I doing on his porch? And he is right to be suspicious of some white guy hanging around pushing pills. The medical profession is as complicit as everyone else in systemic racism. In the past white America has subjected blacks to unethical experimentation, but even now studies show that white doctors systematically under-diagnose and treat African-Americans. There is a simulation experiment presenting hypothetical white and black patients with identical chest pain symptoms. The "objective" evaluations by the doctors lead to 30% fewer referrals for expensive, but life-saving, interventional treatments for black patients. The structure of medical care has always rested in the hands of an elite segment of society. Getting into medical school requires attending a certain slice of colleges, which accept a certain slice of people. Blacks have always been under-represented. Why not be suspicious of me up on the porch, doing my doctor thing?

Medicare is supposed to offer a blanket, equal-access coverage to older Americans. It should be color-blind, and gender-blind and egalitarian. It is not. Patients in Texas receive twice the amount of services of equally sick patients in Oregon. Now, that is not necessarily good, because more medicine is not usually better medicine. But it shows how dramatically different the care under Medicare can be. We often do not really understand why this is the case, but disparity exists, and some of it reflects racial differences.

How could I be different from that racist past? Perhaps I could not, and we are doomed to not trust, and I will not be able to perform as an effective doctor for this woman. But perhaps I can be a person, not a representative of a flawed system. There may still be room for trust between people. Racism's sin is to treat a person as nothing more than a class of people, so the fix might be to treat a person as a person. It will not fix the systematic discrimination of a class, but it could help a single person. I cannot effectively make up for the evils of my class's past: Oregon's ban on African-Americans moving here, Western medicine's power relationship to minority communities. Nope. But I could be authentic on this autumn afternoon. There has to be a level of authenticity available to the earnest and humble. Perhaps not the pure of heart, for that is too high a standard, but at least the hard-working, for that is a standard I do know as a doctor.

We agreed that we would do a short trial of the Parkinsons medication, to see if she felt better and dropped fewer things. I took her blood pressure and listened to her lungs with my stethoscope as the autumn sun stretched the shadows.

As a harried doctor, too full of my own imagined importance, time always stands still for me in this neighborhood. Perhaps it is only my wishful jealousy, but aging usually creates a certain dignity. And these streets, with their peeling paint and poverty, surrounded by an engulfing white culture, ooze dignity. Mrs. J wraps herself in self-respect, forged from I know not what experiences. She speaks so slowly, that even with my one hour visit, I don't have time to hear. Or perhaps I am too afraid to hear. Nobility of spirit can cause fear in the guilty.

Her brother did not return, and I packed my things and left, scheduling a time to visit again in a month. She would forget the appointment, but I knew she would not be far away, and I could always wait on the porch.

Snuffles

"You don't have a soul. You are a soul. You have a body."
--attributed to various 19th century Christian sources

Snuffles is a small Pomeranian dog. His fur is grey and longish and covers his eyes. Like many dogs, he has come to resemble his owner, Karoly. She speaks English nearly impeccably, having immigrated to America in 1966, when she was 19.

"I met my husband and he saved me. My father beat me nearly every day. He was a no-good drunk. My husband took me to America and my mother-in-law was my mother. She told me, You have to stick up for yourself. And I always have, ever since."

“I don’t really want to talk about Germany. But I am stubborn like Germans. And I know how to cook. I still cook a lot, potato salad and casseroles. Those workers across the street, they like my potato salad. I boiled ten pounds of potatoes for them all when we had a potluck when they finished remodeling. And boy, they sure ate that up fast! You never seen anything like that.”

Karoly lives in a one bedroom independent apartment in Lake Oswego. She is bent over, and uses a walker, which does not really fit into her small place, so she leaves it outside the front door, where the squirrels have nibbled on the seat. “I don’t feed them no more, but they come around, you can’t stop them.” Her front yard is a small patch of stone and grass covered with garden gnomes. The cedars overhang the yard and her stoop, dropping needles, and apparently squirrels from time to time.

“I take Snuffles and we walk, around the block and up to the lake sometimes. I’m real active.”

Her small apartment exudes that cloying atmosphere of old smoke. “Oh no, I don’t smoke no more, I might lose this apartment if I smoked! They don’t allow that here. You must be smelling my candles. I quit two years ago.” I just let that comment slide. I am building trust, not calling out her obvious falsehoods and self-delusions. Entering someone’s house implies a significant act of trust. We lock our doors, we put up no soliciting signs, we keep the wide world at bay. But a few people we allow in, and we expect respect in exchange for a view of the sanctum sanctorum. Karoly is 76 and has smoked forever. But she could still have health benefits from stopping, despite the lung and other organ damage already done. Yet, that conversation must wait. Smoking is not just a habit, it is not just a self-medication, it is an aspect of personality. Over the years, the smoking, with its rituals, and shared ceremonies of bonding in the smoking area, becomes an integral part of a person's very being. And not just in some metaphysical form, but actually through changes in receptors and neurotransmitters, up-regulated through years of exposure to nicotine.

Cigarettes shape the soul, for better or worse. Patients may invite me into their house once, to check me out, to evaluate my usefulness. But they don't ask for a surgery on their soul. That takes time. Perhaps an entire lifetime.

People operate on our souls, and my son Noah has been my personal surgeon. At age four he began to have seizures, and soon progressed into intractable epilepsy that no drug could control. He lost his speech, and needs me to help him walk. We assist him with eating, and bathing, and everything in fact. And in return, he provides the meaning in our lives. Noah's seizures appear to have burned out the neural circuitry for the complaint. He exists in the moment, always. He takes each activity for what it offers, which might not be a lot from an outside perspective, but for Noah is enough, and in fact overflowing.

These days I mostly encounter patients "post-operatively", both literally and figuratively. After bodily surgeries we come to houses and check on how people are recovering, whether they have the appropriate follow-up, whether the medications need to be changed. For example, many people with high blood pressure have a neurohumeral response after surgery and do not need their hypertensive medications for a few weeks. If they take their regular pills, they end up with low blood pressure, and feel they have no energy to even get up out of the chair. But mostly, we see people whose souls have been shaped by a lifetime of experience: post-operatively from life's depredations.

Christian theology posits that each person only gets one chance at life, that when the body/soul pairing dies, it awaits an eternal judgment. Other religions opt for multiple chances at a life in this world, with the body perishing, but some sort of soul recycling itself with a reincarnation. How closely the soul is knit to the body seems to determine entirely what might be possible. It has always seemed that the physician, a close observer of both the body and the soul, ought to be able to add some empirical data to this metaphysical debate. But after seeing a lifetime of deaths, we equivocate. At the crucial moment we hesitate, and add nothing.

Karoly continues from her position on the couch, “I had three sons. One lives out in Gresham and drives for Trimet. He takes me places when I need it. But I lost Paul when he was 14. He was killed in 1985.” There is a barely perceptible pause as the central tragedy of her life is spoken, made plain, and passed through, emerging on the other side with a Germanic shrug. “That’s his picture up there, he was a handsome boy.” And indeed he was, a younger blond image of his mother sitting on the sofa, palpably willing him back to life, turning back time to that day when everything changed and she knew with certainty that the universe was indeed as hard as it had always seemed.

How Long Does It Take to Become Indigenous?

"Lewis was an Indian, but he wouldn't say which tribe, only that the lifestyle of Indians east of the Cascades suited him: roaming the land, digging bulbs, living in caves. He didn't live in a cave, of course, although his room in the back of the bowling alley was close enough." -- Heather Bergstrom, Celilo Falls

I find the patient in his small chamber in one of those downtown highrise low-income apartment buildings. "Joe", his name appears listed on the digital lock at the front door; I buzz and he answers, opening the lock remotely from upstairs. On the sixth floor he has an apartment. The door opens to the living room, with a couch, a television and a large friendly golden lab, panting and licking. The dog has taken the entire couch, so we go to the dining nook where there are two chairs. One is his throne, surrounded by his immediate life, within an arm's reach: pill bottles, a small notebook with notations of his blood sugar levels and doctors' instructions, various old cans of soda, an ashtray with old yellow cigarettes, and a few piles of papers of unknown provenance. There is a second chair piled high with dog food. He places it to the side and I sit. We talk.

The nook has a window looking out over downtown Portland, with its freeways and a distant river. Joe clearly does not leave this place very often. His legs are swollen, his lungs wheeze in between cigarettes, and the plump dog does not give up his place on the couch. Meals-on-wheels brings food. He knows his neighbors down the hall. He becomes short-winded with walking a block anyway. This man spent his working life driving a truck on short-haul routes around Oregon, and then finally retiring to his room with a view.

Most medical care requires leaving your home and going into some other building, usually far away. People go to their clinic appointment, or they go to hospitals for more invasive and long-term treatments. The person leaves their house, locks the door behind them and enters a new sterile, artificial world; they assume the label of "patient". As a patient, they receive their procedure or evaluation or medication, and then attempt to return home, to their native habitat, and assimilate the expert recommendation. "Change your diet." "Take this pill." "Stop smoking." "Read these directions." I have come to realize that the "outside expert", that is, me, the doctor, has literally no idea how my advice and treatment affects a life once it returns to its native environment, the home.

Can anyone ever become indigenous again in human history? Or has that moment passed forever? Is our destiny doomed to be a straight arrow, flying forward, leaving the past as a small speck, far behind? Or does history repeat itself in a circle? I get the sense that this man is connected to his place in some fundamental way, perhaps analogous to native peoples. But surely his white skin and European ancestry place him in the category of colonial conqueror rather than First Nation. He enjoyed a white privilege that natives did not. His family story belongs to manifest destiny and the rootless proclamation of "Go west, young man".

And yet... his personal story belongs to this place. Joe could not exist without this block of apartments situated at the end of the Oregon Trail, in the promised land of Portland. And the land is dependent on him as well. "Downtown Portland" as a cultural entity could not exist without this man. There is some reason why the Pearl District, visible down the street from here, became such a desirable spot to live. Part of that reason grows up from the earthy authenticity of poverty, and part from a layer of white guys with dreadlocks and "Che" sweatshirts attracted to that poverty. Joe is characteristic of this region now, and reciprocally he alters the landscape itself. The wealthy, hip, tech-fueled building boom followed here as other white guys were searching for the authenticity that my patients provide.

Joe is now tied inextricably to a small geographical space. Not in a negative way, at least not entirely. His native land has shrunk to a small apartment, a circle of smoking buddies, and a few wet blocks of downtown Portland on the way to the tobacconist. And my job is to try to keep him here. We talk health, and activity and getting out, and how to stay in his apartment safely so he is not forced to move to assisted living somewhere, somewhere far and foreign. Portland has a long history of attempting to create low-income housing, as well as high-density housing. The imperialist myth is that indigenous peoples do not have a history, and that history starts when "civilization" arrives. The erasure of history may be the biggest crime that people can inflict on each other. Modern medicine has certainly created a system that attempts to erase patients' living histories by extracting them from their native habitats and putting them in our sterile, created world of clinics and hospitals.

Swollen legs are not medically dangerous. The medical world calls them "peripheral edema", and they have various causes. Patients and doctors usually leap to the conclusion that the puffiness originates from heart failure. That is, the heart, because it is not pumping strongly enough, does not circulate the usual flow of blood to the kidneys. The kidneys then sense a low-flow state and avidly retain salt and water. Of course, during dehydration or blood loss, this automatic fluid retention would be an adaptive and life-saving response. In the modern world, with its high-salt foods, the fluid retention leads to swollen body parts, such as legs, but sometimes also lungs, where the fluid invades what should be airspaces, and causes difficulty breathing.

But leg edema does not always originate from heart failure. Many people have venous insufficiency where the blood flow down the arteries to the feet and then back is slowed. The "stasis" of blood flow, usually aided by prolonged sitting and dangling the legs, increases pressure in the small veins, and the water component of blood leaks out into the surrounding tissue. Severe edema can even lead to clear fluid "weeping" out from the skin, soaking through stockings and shoes. The circulatory system functions best when the leg muscles contract, helping to squeeze and pump the venous blood back up to the heart. But prolonged sitting without much movement allows pooling and stasis.

Whether caused by heart failure, or by venous insufficiency and immobility, the swollen leg is not dangerous, and many people live their entire lives with large, heavy, elephant legs. But they are uncomfortable, and debilitating, and self-defeating. The more swollen and heavy the legs, the less likely one is to get up and walk, which is the one activity that would help remove the extra fluid. So, we battle the easy chair with dangling legs, where gravity pushes inexorably out until a person oozes down and becomes literally planted to the floor.

We are discussing doses of diuretics, or the water pills that attempt to whip the kidneys into shape and make them eliminate more salt and water, when the apartment door abruptly opens and in steps a tall man in an overcoat. He is rolling a cigarette expertly as he paces back and forth in the small living area. No word is spoken, or introduction made. I am unsure of whether to continue our delicate medical conversation, and pause, hanging between words.

"Umm... so," I am looking back and forth between patient and intruder, both of whom seem oblivious to the other. "Hi!"

The cigarette rolling intruder eyes me suspiciously. He clearly belongs here more than I do. "Who is this guy?" he finally comes out with.

"Hello, I am Dr. Benson." He clearly does not believe a word I am saying and looks over at my patient, still sitting rooted to his chair.

Mr. Tall Cigarette lives down the hall, yet he spends more time in this apartment than his own. Each dwelling here is small on its own, a studio. But together there are hundreds here sharing their lives in this beehive of a building. The neighbors cannot believe that a physician comes in here and helps someone. Most people who enter are enforcing rules or discipline or simply heaping society's abuse onto its low-income citizens. Who is this guy in here, really?

I have interrupted a ritual of visitation that must occur nearly hourly in this rabbit warren of a building. The men sit, brew tea, roll cigarettes, go back and forth between their small chambers, discuss this, discuss that, live and breathe. They all know each other. I imagine they know their downtown blocks, just as I knew the small neighborhood where I grew up for many years in Pullman, Washington. I knew every garbage can and every crooked flagstone path in those few blocks. There was a fence along the back alley where there were two garbage cans stored in a cutout. There was a gap in the fence which would allow a kid to sneak past the cans and cut through from my backyard, across the alley, then through the neighbor's yard and down to the swimming pool. Except for the hound dog on his porch, which could bark, but had never been known to chase past the edge of the yard, and had never bitten anyone -- that we knew of at least. That is the kind of local knowledge of a place that allows one to say they are from there, from that exact block which they know better than anyone else in the world.

There is a limit to the extent of local knowledge and a local sustaining neighborhood. Christopher Robin fixed this limit at 100 acres. Winnie-the-pooh and A. A. Milne's gang of characters stayed within the Hundred Acre Wood which they knew well enough to feel comfortable, and at home, but also large enough to still offer some adventures. Tigger famously gets lost in the woods, and Owl can find a new house in a new tree. And of course, there is always a new bee hive to find, in some unfound tree trunk. In our urban world, 100 acres is about 10 city blocks. I think that's about the right size area to really know, to really know intimately. My childhood memories correspond to that size. The automobile stretches and metastasizes these rules, at the expense of a poverty of real knowledge about the expanded area. I know some streets and some people around Portland, but even a lifetime of this job, visiting people in their little personal 100 acres, would not allow me to know where the daffodils will bloom and which gutter always overflows in the rainstorms.

I suspect becoming indigenous has something to do with limiting one's horizon to a certain place, and thereby deepening one's life. But I don't really know. Instead, I just watch with jealousy as Mr. Tall Cigarette and his friend smoke and make tea.

The Man who Mistook his Life and Just Sat

"If a man has lost a leg or an eye, he knows he has lost a leg or an eye; but if he has lost a self—himself—he cannot know it, because he is no longer there to know it." -- Oliver Sacks, The Man Who Mistook His Wife for a Hat

Mr. S became eligible for concierge home-based care through his Medicare Advantage plan, and his 24 hospital admissions for pneumonia. He was a little proud of this number 24. "I have been in the hospital 24 times for pneumonia," he says with a sincerity bordering on the boastful. "I get sick real quick. Last time I went to my doctor, he gave me a shot in the butt and sent me straight to the emergency department." I looked at the records of these hospital admissions. Some radiographs showed an infiltrate, that is, areas of the lung that should have aerated but were full of pus from the body fighting bacteria. Some of the hospital stays lasted a week, but mostly they were short, just overnight, or two days, with antibiotics and a quick return to health and discharge home.

Medicine has an age-old tradition of doctors relating their most intriguing cases and publishing them for an inquisitive public. Oliver Sacks headlines this tradition and his numerous books should almost be required reading for understanding medicine's golden age, the post World War II boom in clinico-pathological correlation that created modern scientific medicine. In the golden age, the best and the brightest young (nearly entirely) men studied medicine in a few elite institutions. These graduates were then granted medical licenses, a boon of near infinite power, to captain the emerging technological ship of drugs and surgeries. Around this great juggernaut battleship arose a raggle-taggle fleet of support ships: nursing, physical therapy, and so on. But now that we have passed the golden age, we are realizing that maintaining the medical juggernaut may not produce the societal benefit that we had hoped.

The medical battleship has destroyed diseases one by one. And continues to battle those diseases, one by one. Each time Mr. S gets pneumonia, the golden-age medical system springs into action and reduces the enemy to ruins with efficient paramedics, then intensive care ventilators, then broad spectrum antibiotics. Yet the battleship was designed to solve only a certain type of problem, a concrete discrete enemy, such as *Streptococcus pneumoniae* bacteria. Numerous smart subspecialists can all treat particular diseases with remarkable precision: coronary artery plaque rupture, chronic myeloid leukemia, and other such fancy sounding names. Yet, we are finding that success against a disease is not the same as helping a person.

I visited Mr. S in his home a few times and learned about his life. The house was in a newer subdivision in the far eastern suburbs of Gresham. The quiet street had been planned to feel like an older neighborhood, with real sidewalks, and the occasional green space every few blocks. The streets were subtly curved to avoid the impression of conformity. But unlike the more spontaneous neighborhoods one finds in inner southeast Portland, like Hawthorne or Woodstock, the houses here are squashed together, packed in almost. There are trees, but there will never be room for them to attain the grandeur of the queens of Irvington, the monster buckeyes and maples.

There had been a car accident 15 years ago, and Mr. S began having back pain. He never needed surgery on his lower back, and finding old paper records from the pre-computerized days is such a trial, if even possible, that I never was clear on the actual anatomical diagnosis that was assigned at that time. It probably doesn't matter, the result would have been predictably the same: pain medications to help him feel better. Narcotic pain medications. Mr. S has been taking long-acting opiates at least twice daily since that incident. And he still has pain of "7 out of 10" in his lower back.

With chronic pain, Mr. S became less active. He gained weight. He likes to show me his favorite cinnamon rolls. "They come from Smith's, in Vancouver. You've never tasted anything like them." He has an unopened package of four. With a gleam in his eye he describes placing one on a plate, heating it with a pat of butter on top, until it melts and drips down the sides. He developed diabetes, then sleep apnea. The CPAP mask never fit him well, so he still does not use it. His sleep is fitful and he nods off to sleep frequently during the daytime. To stay awake he drinks a RockStar energy shake every day. "Strawberry Cream flavor," he says, "you've never tasted anything like it." Recently he has more stomach bloating, and so was diagnosed with gastroesophageal reflux, and prescribed an acid-blocker medicine. "I still get the bloating," he says, "so I take the medicine twice daily now."

What has always struck me from the many physician case histories that were published, such as Oliver Sacks books, is how intriguing the cases are but how little the doctors actually accomplished. In *The Man who Mistook his Wife for a Hat*, Dr. Sacks masterfully diagnoses agnosia -- inability to recognize faces -- but is powerless to intervene in the patient's life. In fact, he admits that he saw the patient only once! My own Mr. S had certainly been helped by modern medicine. He had been helped too much. Every intervention to "help" one of his diseases had complicated others, and slowly pushed him into a life of amazing medical complication and chronicity. He was complicit in this process, of course. He felt he had received treatment and at each step was taken care of. He was a military veteran, and the idea of equity and fairness in receiving what was due to him in view of his service was important to his identity. He had chosen to take narcotics as they made him feel good. He had chosen his diet. He bore absolutely no resentment against his many fine physicians who had assisted him into his current state of "health". What could be done to intervene in the endless medical cycle of the gentleman? Can we reduce his burden of pneumonia? Can we keep him awake in the day and able to sleep at night? Can he enjoy his meals and not suffer from bloating?

Mr. S is at greatest risk from his numerous cases of pneumonia. He has been lucky, but pneumonia can kill, at any age. Let's start with 24 cases of pneumonia and unpack the multiple medical issues. First, pneumonia so many times is truly unusual. The body has a series of defenses to prevent bacteria in the lungs: nasal filtration of incoming air, with immune cells lining the passages. Then the entire respiratory passage produces mucus to entrap particles and bacteria, and microscopic hair on cells, the cilia, constantly beats to move foreign particles up and out of the lungs and throat. Finally, the thin air exchange tissue deep in the lungs is surrounded by blood vessels that bring fresh infection-fighting white cells, to every section of the lung. So, were these 24 hospital admissions all actually pneumonia? When a patient arrives in the emergency department with a fever, breathing fast, and lab tests that indicate infection, doctors often assume pneumonia and treat it, because the alternative of doing nothing until one can be certain, is too dangerous. The infection could worsen quickly, causing organ failure and death.

If these were all, or mostly, pneumonia admissions, why did some resolve so quickly, even overnight? Pneumonia usually has a multi-day course, worsening for a few days before reaching its crisis and then slowly improving over the course of ten days or more. Mr. S had experienced a few episodes like that, but most were much faster. There are immune deficiencies that can worsen pneumonia, such as immunoglobulin deficiencies. These would likely have showed up much earlier in his life, not when he turned 60. Other lung diseases can predispose to pneumonia, such as emphysema. And indeed he was smoker for many years, and the CT scans of his lungs show pockets of air, bullae, that indicate destruction of surrounding tissue. The bullae do not exchange oxygen well, thus the air hunger of this disease, and they leave pockets where bacteria can grow without an intimate web of capillaries to supply infection-fighting white cells. But even with emphysema, 24 bouts of pneumonia is a lot.

He was suspicious that anything that the VA and other doctors had given him could actually be worsening his condition and causing pneumonia. For months I visited and slowly convinced him to try tapering off the acid blocking medicine. Then we worked on reducing the narcotics. He is more awake during the days now. And he has not had a single bout of pneumonia.

22 Years in 300 Square Feet Under the Cedars

> *"It is not quite true that you can't go home again. I have done it, coming back here. But it gets less likely. We have had too many divorces, we have consumed too much transportation, we have lived too shallowly in too many places." --Wallace Stegner, Angle of Repose*

The urban density of Portland's Pearl district gradually decreases away from the center as you travel east or west. The deliberate urban planning of the core thins into deliberately unplanned areas that have been settled, or unsettled, by those seeking inexpensive options and others simply looking for freedom. For the most part, freedom equates with an RV.

The RV is the modern symbol of Western freedom. And of Western poverty. Those who have become hemmed in by their jobs and lifestyles choose RVs to reconnect with that open-road feeling that brought them to the west in the first place. And then they park when they tire of their rootless Arizona winter get-away. Others choose, or fall into, the RV lifestyle permanently. They park out on the periphery of Portland, off the main roads, where the old growth cedars hide them from view, where nobody complains about the rusting Chevrolet out back, where anything goes. I visit such a collection of recreational vehicles near Sandy. You could live in Portland your whole life and never find this place. You could never imagine this place, quiet - almost tomb-like - under the slow drip of the canopy. Out here, RV stands for Readily aVailable housing. I am visiting a couple who tell me they have lived here for 22 years.

The road forms a circle, with "campsites" placed along the outer spokes. Each site guards its metal-sided house, a small enclosure with wheels. Or at least with axles. Most of the wheels have been removed to serve other purposes, on other vehicles that might actually roll somewhere. These campsites house only tin boxes where the temporary has become permanent.

Joe and his wife live here, and have lived here in this RV for 22 years. They added a porch at some point, doubling the livable area, at least in the summer. Inside the flimsy door, the living space is "cozy", or "jammed", depending on how you see it. The layout of a table, a kitchenette and back bedroom with bath is what one might call "efficient". In fact, with only four spots for a human body in the home, the permutations of travel between table and the 3 other spots are limited. The carpet shows the worn deer trails.

Joe is just back from the hospital where he was admitted with chest pain. He has severe coronary artery disease and gets chest pains all the time. He smoked for nearly the entire 22 years he has lived in this RV. Until a few months ago when he had a large myocardial infarction -- a heart attack. One of the partially blocked arteries that surround the outside of the heart and supply the heart muscle itself with blood and oxygen, ruptured on its inside wall. The normally smooth lining had decayed and roughened over the years, from the effects of cigarettes and cholesterol. The frayed lining then attracted the bloodstream's natural clotting agents, and within minutes the artery clotted closed, blocking oxygen to the heart muscle. His face turned ashen and he started sweating, feeling like he could not catch his breath. It takes even an ambulance a while to find this place, out off the beaten path. But he got to the hospital where a stent was skillfully threaded up through an artery from the groin, up ever larger arteries to the top of the heart, where the coronary arteries branch off, and then into the area of blockage. When the cardiologist inflates the balloon inside the artery, and the stent opens the artery, the pain can resolve nearly instantly.

But now Joe is home again, and facing some changes. There are new medications. There are inhalers for the lung disease. There are pages of instructions and advice on diet, and exercise, and regimens for pills. There is everything that is antithetical to a lifetime living in an RV. There is no more freedom. Some people are free and then die, but most people are free and then not free so much. Just like me, I was never as free as I thought I could be. There was always the next big trip I was going to take, the next wilderness area to hike. Instead I have a disabled son Noah and my exploration and freedom have shrunk. The idea of the RV and American West tempt me daily. The lack of a full-size bathroom to deal with incontinence after seizures quickly stops these daydreams.

The West as an idea is all about freedom. Everything that is America, is the West, only more so. I understand this man parking his RV amongst the cedars because it was the free-est place he could imagine. Everyone sought freedom going west, and everyone arrived at the end of their imaginations. It is our national mythology, expressed in metallic form. Europeans fleeing tyranny came here to new lands they could fashion and mold to express their human creations. And 500 years later we see the results of this human fashioning, having remade the west into an image of ourselves. The road west ends near Portland, under a tree, where the RV is rusting, and the sick man has never taken a walk around his campground, under the cedars. He is too sick, having smoked his lungs out.

"I sold RVs for years," he relates when we sit and talk. "Can you believe it? I worked at a dealership. People come in, they want an RV, I sold it to 'em. It was a good job. The dealership is just down the road."

I can believe it, for this is the spiritual home of the recreational vehicle. Some might argue that Arizona is the true birthplace of this uniquely American creation, but I argue for Oregon; Arizona is simply the site of the pilgrimage. Oregon, as the end of the westward trail, and the logical end of Manifest Destiny, is where the RV succeeded where the Conestoga wagon could not: to ensure permanent rootlessness. Not far from here sits the End of the Oregon Trail Museum. An oxymoron, for there is no end to the Oregon Trail, and this campground proves it. Manifest Destiny always implied that "farther" was necessarily better, and by implication, that means that "more" is also to be preferred.

Modern medicine also follows manifest destiny in preferring more intervention and treatment. There is a well-known bias in publishing clinical trials that have positive results compared to publishing trials that have negative results. Studies that show that interventions do not work, do not help the patient, are 10 times less likely to get published in respectable journals and read by other doctors. Who wants to read about failure? And how can a failed treatment advance an academic career? So, we perpetuate the myth that we are continually advancing and creating meaningful improvements in medicine all the time. The reality is not that we make no significant medical advances, but that they take a lot more investment and time then the public realizes.

Cardiac care is an area that has seen remarkable improvement over the course of the last 50 years. From the 1920's science realized that "heart attacks" were caused by blockages in the arteries that surround the outside of the heart muscle and supply it with its blood, oxygen and nutrients, thereby depriving sections of the muscle and killing them, creating a scar on the heart. Then came the realization that these clots in the arteries were caused by cholesterol plaques building up in the walls of the arteries, and then rupturing and exposing their rough surfaces which then attract clotting elements, quickly closing the artery. And slowly we have learned what factors make these artery walls more likely to rupture: high fat diets, smoking, lack of exercise, some genetic factors. Finally, we developed ways of reopening closed arteries by opening metal cages, or stents, in the blocked areas. Survival from heart attacks has risen considerably, from the 1950's when we thought that because the heart muscle was damaged it should be "rested" with weeks of bedrest, to now.

Given our predilection for interpolating into the future, we have assumed that since heart attacks are caused by blocked arteries, and stents fix blocked arteries, we should stent open every spot that is blocked. It makes intuitive sense. And it keeps cardiologists employed, doing complex technical procedures in expensive sterile catheterization labs in hospitals. We have wonderful imaging tests that can find partially blocked arteries, so-called "stress tests" that take pictures of the heart and show which regions are not getting full blood flow. Anyone with a twinge of chest pain has had such stress tests, usually numerous times in their lives. Once a plaque is found, the whole establishment swings into action, and nearly painlessly a stent is placed. Patients feel that something exciting and high-tech has been done to save their lives. Hospitals and doctors also feel good, hopefully not just because of the large billing opportunity.

A few pioneering studies have started to show that more interventions do not always mean better care, however. In the middle of a heart attack, an acutely blocked artery, everyone agrees that stenting is best. But for people with partial blockages, of which it turns out that almost all of us have some, simply improving diet, exercise, and a few old-school medications to lower cholesterol, produce the same or better outcomes than the stents. In other words, by reversing all the unhealthy behaviors that cause lipid buildup, we can reverse the disease and chest pains actually go away, without any high-tech interventions such as coronary stents. This result is not widely known amongst the public, and is greeted with much skepticism amongst my patients. Less is not more out here, which corresponds to our entire experience of the "west".

The American west is just like the rest of America, "only moreso". The west, with its sublime landscapes and soaring peaks, has always reflected our unique ideology of "moreso". More is better, farther west is better, farther down the trail is better, bigger cars are better. The west is America's superlative. And we're proud of it. So we want cardiac stents, and a whole bunch of other medical treatments. I have encountered a few patients over the years who prefer less treatment. They are a rare breed, at least for doctors. Those who do not want medical interventions tend to avoid doctors and their clinics, and so we never meet these people, who surely exist out on the fringes somewhere, happily cultivating their own gardens. This in itself is a horrible indictment of my profession. We have become labelled and stereotyped as pill-pushers and surgery sharks. The wise avoid us and park their RVs on the other side of the street.

The ultimate symbol of Western freedom circles around and becomes the final prison. The western wilderness paradises that harbor the fleets of campers become their own ghettos. The inhabitants achieve the pinnacle of rootless freedom by becoming trapped in their little tin boxes. I love the irony of the west for it shows the irony of medicine. We devote ourselves to a healing profession to preserve human freedom, yet with every treatment we tie our patients inexorably into the net of the medical system. Will I ever create an authentic healing practice out here at the end of road? Have we driven too many miles and climbed to the tops of all the peaks? Will we eventually accept less because we are exhausted from it all, or will the drip, drip from the cedar boughs yet uncover some balance of place and perspective?

Last Night They Had This Guy Dying

"Can you cough it up loud and strong
The immigrants, they wanna sing all night long
It could be anywhere
Most likely could be any frontier...
Straight to hell boy
Go straight to hell boy"
--The Clash, "Straight to Hell"

"I wish they would finish that construction next door. They came in here and replaced my window. I told them that they should talk to their guys because they stand around an awful lot. I was a contractor and I never let my workers stand around like that. They had to work if they wanted to get paid. And they don't do a good job now like we used to. Look out there at the building wrap, that yellow covering, just open like that! It's flapping in the wind! Why don't they finish it and put the siding on, so it matches everything else? The buildings around here are white, with some brown trim. Can't they see that? The yellow stuff just moves around in the wind. I see it out the window. Every time the breeze comes by I see that yellow move out the window. The wind blows, the yellow moves. The wind blows, the yellow moves. And those guys just stand around. I've seen them, sometimes on their phones. Do they pay those guys? I pay to live here and it's not cheap, let me tell you. Then they pay these workers out of that? What a waste! They don't work like we used to. They're not even workers, really. They are just lookers.

"I don't mean to be racist, but they have these Mexicans here. She is 4 foot 10 or so, she just does not talk like the others and I don't know what she is doing. Every night they come in to help me get to bed. It's not complicated. It's simple. I like it done right. First, move my pillows from the chair to the bed, then get my slippers so I'm ready to stand... But the Mexican can't get it right. She gets the slippers first. I hate it."

"I just don't sleep well. I keep the door open about 6 inches. Then I can see some light out in the hall but it's not too noisy. This place isn't like home. But I can't manage on my own anymore. Most of the people are good, but not those Mexicans. I don't mean to be racist, but they just don't talk like the others so they don't know what they are doing.

"I lie awake at night a lot. Yeah, I think about my wife. I had a dream that she was having an affair. She's been dead 3 years now. I woke up and knew it wasn't true. I knew it wasn't true when I saw the crack of light coming in past the door. We didn't live here when she was alive. We had a house. And some roses in the front yard. She used to trim them every year. I don't know why I would think she was having an affair. But I woke up. I always wake up. It keeps coming back to me and I think about it.

"I had another dream. I was trying to complete a house. We were framing it up, the whole crew. Back then we used hammers not these fancy nail guns. Those are just for lazy people. Pop, pop, pop and they think they have worked a whole day. Well, we swung a hammer. Each guy carried his own hammer and that was something, hanging there by your side, that felt good there by your side. In the dream the walls kept falling down. I screamed at those guys, don't you know how to put in a nail? We would nail the framing up, but it just kept falling over. And then I screamed at them again. Man, I used to get good workers, but those guys couldn't even put a nail in straight! I chewed them out good, real good. Then I started swinging my hammer around. Yeah, then I fell off that damn house! I didn't hit the ground. Damn! I guess that was just a dream, wasn't it?

"I like my TV on. I know you've told me to turn it off and I might sleep better. But I like it! Stuff happens on that TV. Nothing happens here in my room. I want to see what's happening. I know I'm old, but I should get to know what's happening. They had this guy on TV who was shooting people. He was walking down the street, all dark outside, there weren't even any streetlights, I don't know why. And no cars either I guess. It was just an empty street, real dark. No one was around, just this guy shooting people. I mean... I guess there were people he was shooting around then? Well, maybe there weren't any people. I guess maybe that was a dream too, wasn't it?

"Why am I having all these dreams, doc? I think these helpers must have talked to you because they keep turning off my TV at night, just like you said. Even that Mexican, she turns it off too. Then she sang for me. She has a real nice voice. I didn't know the words, some Mexican song I guess. I didn't know those Mexicans had such nice songs! You know I directed the choir at church? Maybe she knows that? I would have liked to have her in my choir, she really has a voice. Was that a dream? No, I think she did sing. Some of them sing at night for me. Some of them do. Even that chaplain who comes by, we have been singing together. I can't read from the hymnal much now. I guess I still remember those hymns anyway, don't I? I think I slept that night.

"Last night they had this guy dying down the hall. What a commotion. I should have closed my door last night. I don't know why they needed all that bother. Their voices were loud. That Mexican girl came in, at least she was quiet. She didn't tell me what was going on, but I didn't care. He was dying. I wish they would be quieter with that. Who wants to listen to a guy dying?

"He must have died because eventually it all quieted down. But I still couldn't sleep. When will I die? I think about that a lot."

Tom Still Has Diarrhea

"Every element of the cosmos has a place in the family. Everything is alive and has needs and rights. Therefore people must concern themselves with the health and wellbeing of everything in the cosmos..."
--Susan A Miller, Native Historians Write Back

"How was Charlie Jones?" our nurse care manager asks as I pass through our administrative office one morning.

"Ummm..." I mumble, mind racing. The name recalls nothing for me. Did I just see this patient? "Remind me what that was about?"

She looks at me with a resigned expression, "The one you saw yesterday who was complaining of pain in his shoulder and chest."

Still nothing, no patient pops into my head, no house I had visited, no cluster of symptoms and treatments that I had recommended.

“Did I see him?”

My team is used to this with me. While I interact with a patient, everything else leaves my concentration and I focus on entirely on that particular patient. But later I recall nothing, my attention moving on to the next story. Except if I think about the place.

“He lives out in Oregon City, and you had to go out of your way in the afternoon to get down there.”

Instantly, a thin man who lives up long narrow stairs in an apartment that overlooks a stand of spruce jumps into my consciousness. As does his medical history of lung cancer treated by surgical resection, and his subsequent weight loss. He struggles with eating an adequate diet living on his own. And he is afraid of every little twinge in his body, that it might signify a return of cancer or some other mortal malady. For me, geography functions as the placeholder in my memory for nearly everything.

I drive around Portland’s neighborhoods and people flash before me. Tommie who just went on hospice at the taco stand on SE 102nd Avenue. Mrs. Philomen with a recurrence of colon cancer at the nondescript corner of N Detroit and N Jessup. The chronic pain that dominates a living room window with the sweeping view east over downtown from SW Slavin Road.

I first learned about the power of geography over people at one of my first jobs, long before medical school, working for Pacific Crest Outward Bound. During college summers I helped lead wilderness expeditions up and down the mountains of the west, from Joshua Tree to Kings Canyon, up to the Sisters Wilderness and Mt. Adams. Outward Bound had various outdoors programs but I worked in the "hoods in the woods" division where we took juvenile delinquents from the city on month-long expeditions far out into the wilderness, teaching rock climbing, glacier travel, and self-worth. I started out in charge of logistics, packing the gear and shuttling it to the trailheads to await the bus that brought wide-eyed kids out from town to this new foreign country at the end of a dirt road.

At the trailhead a group of self-conscious kids would step down from their known world of the city, and enter our known world, the wilderness. Still trying to look cool, these teenagers would negotiate the mud and the sap, stripping off their hoodies and donning our fleece and vibram boots. Over the next weeks, each one would encounter his or her inner crisis at a different point. I sat with one boy as he anxiously chewed the top of his walking stick while thunder boomed around us at a campsite on Bear Creek in the Goat Rocks Wilderness.

Another one met his limit as we set up tents on a snowfield on the north slope of Mt. Adams, realizing that the empty mountain could swallow his anger and not strike back at him. We always ended the month-long course with a six mile run to meet the parents on the last day. Ronnie, the smallest one, the timid one, finished the whole run and fell, smiling, into is parents' arms, having completed something finally, having gained a sense of himself. These mountains speak, and their language can be heard by anyone who spends enough time in them.

The trails and peaks of the west are marked in my memory with the experiences that those beautiful landscapes have etched into me and into others. I grew up in those summers and became a man by watching the transformation of place on people. Sometimes the smallest part of the land did its magic, like the time we had to do a stream crossing by boulder-hopping with heavy packs, and one boy simply was too scared. The rest of the group went ahead while I talked him through it and over it. His life changed forever at that moment, there at that small 10 foot area, on an obscure trail, just roaring water and hard rock. It doesn't take a beautiful panoramic view, or a famous waterfall to change your life forever. Every little place changes us daily.

As I drive through Tom's neighborhood I pass the high fence separating the building's parking from the neighborhood church. It is, absurdly, painted orange, and is wilting in the Oregon humidity, slowly decaying and turning itself back into brown dirt, plank by plank. This is the "Tom street" and every detail of his medical history lives in its straightness, the cutout curb leading past the sagging fence into the parking lot surrounded by military green apartment buildings. I pull in over the speed bumps and park. I return to Tom's basement apartment and it is still raining. The water has leaked through the patio door so now the rug is rolled up in the kitchen. But Tom is not laying curled up on the couch; he is dressed and has had a haircut. But he is still angry.

His last visit to the gastroenterologist resulted in yet a new possible diagnosis for his diarrhea: Irritable Bowel Syndrome. This is a relatively common and benign condition where the nerve cells of the gut fire spontaneously, causing contractions and diarrhea. Or occasionally the opposite, no gut muscle contraction at all and complete constipation. But it is a "syndrome", which means science does not really understand what causes it, so we just label a cluster of symptoms. There are many syndromes in medicine. There are so many areas where our physiological knowledge is incomplete, but we know that certain groups of symptoms are related and all caused by one thing. Down syndrome. Raynaud syndrome. And my own son's disease, Lennox-Gastaut syndrome.

The label of "syndrome" conjures up the unstated truism of incomplete scientific knowledge. With this lack of firm, confirmed knowledge, the door also opens to speculation, and alternative explanations. Alternative medicine and outright quackery exploit this incompleteness by proposing their own explanations: obscure toxicities, nutrition deficits, or even spirits and "humors." Who is to say their alternative explanations are wrong when science does not know the answer itself? If you can't explain it, then your explanations must be wrong, goes the thinking.

The fallacy here is that incomplete knowledge shows a deficit in science. In fact, the opposite is true. Science is more about recognizing the limits of human knowledge than asserting bold new truths. Only by using a scientific method can we ever come to the realization that we do not know something. Only this much I know, and nothing more, is what the result of every study proclaims. The syndrome in medicine is just such an assertion, that we simply do not yet understand the physiologic factors producing the signs and symptoms that we see.

Unfortunately, humans like to have explanations, and are rarely satisfied with statements of lack of knowledge. This is where speculative alternative medicine, pseudo-science and internet quackery are able to flourish. Who is to say that their alternative explanations aren't correct when you don't know what is correct? For the ill and desperate, this argument can go a long way. It can take you to the local herb shop or all the way to a "stem cell lab in Mexico" that promises a cure to all that ails you. Unfortunately, for all that science does not know, it knows what it does not know, and we arrive at our hard-fought knowledge through many, many negative studies. We know a lot about what does *not* work, even if we often don't know what *will* work for a certain disease.

We really do not know what causes Irritable Bowel Syndrome. The nervous system controlling the intestines remains a mystery. And so the speculators are out there, feeding off the enigma. It must be a food allergy, it must be an infection, it must be repressed childhood trauma. I have watched Tom in the throes of his cramping diarrhea. He sweats, he is in pain, he is pale and miserable. I have also seen other irritable bowel patients, where the cramping and diarrhea are more annoying than life-altering. These symptoms seem severe to me and my 20 years of experience. So I leave my mind open to the possibility that this represents more than just irritable bowel. This could still be carcinoid, or it still could be narcotic withdrawal. Sometimes it is good not to know. Time will pass. We don't have to act at every moment. Diseases will declare themselves. The hardest advice to give can be "let's watch and wait and do nothing now."

When we wait, we let the underlying disease process interact with the patient, without disturbance. The basement apartment, the military green paint, the falling fence, the spring rain... all these and more will produce a result. Tom is not in danger of imminent death. We can wait and let the wilderness speak, let the mountains produce their result. This unique combination of person, place and circumstances needs to play itself out. Perhaps Tom's long-lost sister will show up and tip the balance? Perhaps the summer sunshine will work its magic even down in a basement apartment? The factors that we do not understand will always outnumber the ones that we do. The mask of the healer hates syndromes. So I take off the mask and drive to a different neighborhood.

The Finer Fruits

"Most men, even in this comparatively free country, through mere ignorance and mistake, are so occupied with the factitious cares and superfluously coarse labors of life that its finer fruits cannot be plucked by them." -- Henry David Thoreau, Walden

The Conrads had just returned from Florida where they went on a cruise with their grandkids. At our last visit in the fall, they had been planning this trip which Phyllis was unsure if she would have the energy for since completing her chemotherapy for lymphoma. Lymphoma is a cancer of the immune system cells. The cells continuously monitor our own bodies for invading bacteria and viruses. The cells concentrate in small "nodes" placed strategically around the entry points for pathogens, such as the throat and nose, and the intestines. The cells are pre-programmed to recognize threats and then quickly multiply themselves to fight those threats. This ability to rapidly multiply becomes dangerous when the cells themselves become altered with cancer.

Just back from their dream vacation, Phyllis lay ill on the couch, vomiting uncontrollably. "I just had to go... We had to go. It was worth it. All the grandkids were there! All of them!" She looked ill and pale against the red couch, covered by a white blanket. "The last day on the ship I felt a little queasy, but it was rocking in the water. A lot of people didn't quite feel right."

"When did you start throwing up?" I ask as I start typing on the laptop, documenting in her chart. In the evenings and on weekends, we respond to more urgent needs from our cohort of patients. The boundary between doing okay and becoming ill is short and sharp with a long medication list and multiple illnesses. Catching illness early is part of how we keep people at home.

"Not until I got home, after the flight. That was three days ago. I just can't keep anything down. I try to drink but I vomit. It's mostly bile now."

"Have you been dizzy or lightheaded?"

"Yes," she continues, "since the beginning my head just hasn't felt right."

Dizziness is the most vexing medical symptom because it is so non-specific and can stem from something as benign as overexertion to diseases as severe as a brainstem stroke. It often helps to clarify what is meant by "dizzy": an internal sensation of imbalance, or vertigo which implies actual movement of the visual field. Phyllis has atrial fibrillation, where the upper chambers of the heart do not beat regularly and instead quiver, causing an irregular heartbeat and irregular blood flow, predisposing to blood clots which can travel from the heart to the brain and cause a stroke. Or perhaps the lymphoma has returned, either in the intestines or sometimes surrounding the brain? Or more likely, she has simply been exposed to one of the innumerable gut viruses that multiply quickly and are incredibly easy to transmit in the closed spaces of a cruise ship.

We complete a thorough neurological exam, which finishes by having her stand. "Now put your arms out and close your eyes." She closes them without affecting her balance at all. She is not even swaying. Then, with her eyes still closed and without warning her, I push her forward from the upper back, ready with my other hand to catch her if she loses balance.

"Hey!" she startles but only sways an inch before recovery. It's a trick test of course. I need to know if her brainstem and posterior columns of the spine are intact and able to unconsciously sense the motion without the inputs of the eyes, recovering balance by sending the appropriate movement signals out to the body.

"I'm sorry, but I can't warn you about the push, or you might be able to consciously anticipate, throwing off the test. But no worries, everything seems fine, from your stomach to your brain. I think you just got a stomach bug." It's a generic term for any virus or bacteria or bacterial toxin that she could have ingested on her travels. The treatment is the same for all of them, whether she got it from spoiled food or a sick grandchild: nothing. Antibiotics don't help these episodes. Performing numerous sophisticated tests of the stool to identify the culprit does not help except in a few rare cases. The body vomits or has runny stool to wash out the culprit, and then heals, on its own.

"You are going to be fine. But let's make sure you don't get dehydrated. I'll put in an IV and we'll give you some fluids and some nausea medicine."

She lies back on the couch and I kneel by her side, preparing my equipment. The process is simple, and performed by nurses, not doctors in most medical situations. Find a likely vein, put an elastic around the upper arm to engorge and plump up the vein. Swab the site with some alcohol, take the cap off the needle inside its soft rubber catheter sheath. Stabilize the vein with the other hand, talking softly about something else to distract the patient from the upcoming sharp poke. This is a ritual in and of itself, performed thousands of times daily around the world in healthcare. It is the ritual which defines admission into the hidden world inside the body, the mysterious world under the skin which the initiated, the doctors and nurses, have access to but the uninitiated, the public, do not.

The needle slides smoothly under the skin. With the slight flash of pain and redness within the catheter hub, the patient feels better immediately, for they know that all the magic of modern medicine is now accessible. We enter the inscrutable world of the vein, the domain of the high-tech which symbolizes the weight of scanners, white coats and sterile fields. I push the rubber catheter forward and withdraw the sharp needle, retracting and locking it away as I place it into the sharp waste disposal. I attach the IV tubing and the fluids start to drip through the catheter and into the body. This is simply salt water, but it carries the weight of expectations.

Medical students occasionally start an IV or hook up tubing as part of their training, but afterwards doctors only give orders. It would be rare indeed in a hospital or clinic for the provider to "waste their time" with these routine tasks. Nurses accomplish the actual care of patients; doctors just determine what that care should be. Patients are not admitted to hospitals in order to get the care of doctors. They are admitted in order to get the care of nurses, who will clean and bathe and give medications and treatments. But here, I get the satisfaction of doing the nursing care. Somehow priming the tubing, pulling the syringe back to draw up the medicine, using my thumb to click the stop wheel, these mundane tasks feel more important than all my cerebral interpretations of x-rays and lab results.

Gravity assists the fluid to run down into the vein, but I don't carry the ubiquitous hospital IV pole with me on my home visits. So we place the bag of fluid up on portable clothes hanger rack they have. Phyllis relaxes back as the nausea medicine, the fluids, and the ritual take their effect. I sit next to her on the chair, charting in my computer as silence surrounds us in the house. Is it my imagination, or do the lines in her face seem to be softening? Her color returns as she sleeps.

Why can't medicine always be this easy? When my son Noah seizes and can't eat at home, why can't I cure him this effortlessly? A clock ticks in the background on this Saturday afternoon as tears come to my eyes. I want this medical ritual to work for me too, for my family too. But it doesn't, and it won't. Soon this timeless moment where a doctor is of some use will end. I will get a text from home, telling me of a seizure, and I will rudely return to real life.

A Breath of Fresh Air

"The real purpose of the scientific method is to make sure nature hasn't misled you into thinking you know something you actually don't know." – Robert Pirsig, Zen and the Art of Motorcycle Maintenance.

Exit 17 from I-205 descends off the overpass into Lents and the Johnson Creek drainage. On a spring day with the windows down, the biting odor of marijuana inevitably greets me. The smell of weed is a Portland institution by now. Legalization and a long-standing culture, as well as a miraculous growing season, has blossomed into a world of bud. And nowhere more than Johnson Creek, a fertile drainage which has somehow produced more used car lots than nurseries. Two lefts and a right and I cross the Springwater Trail and head into a neighborhood of small working-class houses where I have a lot of patients who can't breathe.

Today I park beside the low chain-link fence holding back a fiercely barking dog and knock at the place next door. Most of these houses hold retirees, and when you have chronic obstructive pulmonary disease, it is a chore to get out of the house and go very far. Mrs. J__ does not get up from her chair in the corner of the living room when I enter. She is recovering from a recent bout of exacerbation of her chronic obstructive pulmonary disease, and moving around is difficult. She sits perched on her chair, with oxygen tubing draped from nose to ears and down across the floor to a concentrator in the other room. Two liters per minute, continuous, to supplement the 21% that the Earth itself supplies.

Emphysema and COPD, which are essentially the same disease, involve the destruction of the supporting tissue surrounding the microscopic airways. Overwhelmingly, but not universally, this destruction is caused by cigarette smoke, with its wicked brew of chemicals, killing these cells one by one over the years, with each lungful. Without supportive connective tissue, the airways collapse, and big cavities, or "bullae" appear. The miniature arteries and miniature air passages are no longer touching and can no longer exchange oxygen and carbon dioxide. The air goes in and out, but the person can no longer "breathe" because they aren't exchanging gases. The oxygen level in the blood goes down, and the carbon dioxide level goes up. So the person compensates by trying to suck more in with each breath, and by breathing faster. The chest volume slowly expands and many people with this disease develop "barrel chests," and pursed-lip breathes in an attempt to increase the pressure inside the lungs and keep the airways open so they don't collapse. Breathing that deeply and that fast requires bigger and bigger muscles so often COPD produces enlarged strap muscles of the neck, contracting with each breath to try to pull the lungs open. And people start to lose weight, as the work of breathing takes over a greater and greater proportion of their efforts. As COPD becomes "end-stage", the body becomes a breathing machine. The arms are used to prop up the chest and keep the lungs open. The heart pumps faster and harder to push blood through the collapsed passages of the lung. All the fat and muscle reserves of the body get converted into energy for the lung muscles to use, incessantly pushing and pulling, in and out, out and in, you can never stop breathing, not even for a moment.

Becoming a breathing machine is not a pleasant process. Humans are not built to be single-purpose machines, but instead well-rounded living creatures who eat, drink, laugh and run. As the disease progresses, these other activities fall slowly to the wayside, one by one, as breathing takes over the body, and eventually the preoccupation of the mind. It can be no other way, for we are alive and must breathe, and our body systems will do whatever it takes so we keep breathing, even if that means taking over the brain so that we think of nothing else but breathing. In and out, out and in, in and out. You cannot talk to someone having an exacerbation of their COPD about anything else but their breathing. They simply cannot concentrate on any other subject. The lungs have taken over every other organ, including the brain. "I must have air, I must have air," are the signals from the lowered blood oxygen level, and there is nothing more primal than that signal. It is the signal of the newborn who gasps and fills her lungs for the first time, and then wails. It is the signal from the bottom of the pool as you try to stay down longer and beat your friends at the breath-holding contest. The imperious corporeal command to breathe stems from each cell's requirement to have oxygen to receive the electrons, as they cascade down the molecular chain, creating energy for the cell's functions. We are an oxygen-dependent species in an oxygen-dependent world, and breath is life.

Mrs. J___ perches on the edge of her chair, leaning forward a little. Her chest rises with each breath, the shoulders rise, pulling open the chest so air can enter the lungs. With each exhalation, she purses her lips together just a little. This is an adaptation that most people with obstructive lung disease eventually take on, actually preventing the easy passage of air out of the lungs by narrowing the mouth and lips. The narrowed upper airway increases the air pressure down into the lungs and helps splint open the damaged tissues that otherwise would collapse with the extra pressure required to exhale. It is called "pursed lip breathing" and is so helpful that it is taught in pulmonary rehabilitation classes. But it's a lot of work. Every breath is a lot of work. Rather than smoothly sliding in and out, Mrs. J___'s breath rattles and shimmies. It wheezes and moans. The body has an imperceptible shake twenty times a minute. That lung-burning ache that athletes get with maximal exertion, Mrs. J___ has that all the time, just sitting.

I was told that Mrs. J___ suffered from anxiety, by the nurse who had spoken with her earlier, and that she wanted something to help with that. To be honest, I have never met someone with obstructive lung disease who does *not* have anxiety. Anxiety is the sensation of a lack of ease, of something bad imminently about to occur. This is sort of the definition of not being able to breathe. Ease of breath is what defines the calmness of yoga and meditative practice, just as the inability to breathe is what defines anxiety.

"Have you used your nebulizer today?" I begin our conversation.

"Yes... I have... I got it... from the... bedroom... and brought it... out here..." Speaking normally actually requires a remarkable reserve of respiratory capacity that we usually take for granted. Getting through a sentence or two of verbal output without pausing to take a breath is actually an amazing accomplishment and many of my patients can't do it. I recall one late night during my residency, rounding in the intensive care unit with the pulmonologist. "The lung is the master organ," he said, likely in exactly the tone of voice that one can imagine such a statement would be uttered by an expert. Ultimately we define death as what occurs when the heart stops, not the lung, but the heart doesn't really control anything else. The heart beats and organs get their blood supply; it's just a pump, and can be replaced mechanically by CPR and bypass machines. Not so with the lung. First, the narrow tube of the airway from the mouth and nose to the lungs is a constant issue: it gets blocked, food goes down it, it swells up, it gets clogged with mucus. Those six inches of mucous-lined soft passage has a whole specialty dedicated just to it: anesthesia. Next, the exchange of oxygen and carbon dioxide actually determines the acid-base balance of the blood and all the body tissues through a complex pathway involving bicarbonate that vexes all medical students. And finally, the lung tissue is essentially a micron thick membrane between the outside world, with its dirt and pathogens, and the sterile clean blood supply. What could go wrong?

Mrs. J___ has 2 to 3 word dyspnea, a euphemism for only being able to say a few words before needing to pause again for breath. The scary part is that this is her baseline. She has this all the time. She has had all the treatments, she uses 3 inhalers and her nebulizer machine multiple times per day. She is not going to get better. The chronic damage of COPD occasionally flares up into "exacerbations" where the bacteria in the lungs multiply, the mucous production increases, the smooth muscle around the microscopic air passages tighten, and wheezing and coughing begin. Almost anything can bring this on with fragile lungs: viruses, pollen, wind, cold. Sometimes we can calm down the acute inflammation by giving some antibiotics and steroids. Anyone with bad COPD has had multiple courses of prednisone, or eventually even chronic prednisone, a dose every day to try to calm down the angry tissues lining the air passages. Prednisone has side effects of redistributing fat on the body, causing a hump on the upper back, and flattening the face.

She uses three regular inhaled medications. They open the airways, decrease the mucous production, and have prolonged her life. The ads on television for these medications portray young-appearing women playing happily with grandkids in a flowery meadow. This is the image we all want to form of how medicine will help us: it will take us from suffering to some sort of Edenic paradise of family and love. These inhalers have saved

Mrs. J___'s life, but they don't deliver a field in summer. For the most part they deliver more of what you already have. They deliver a prolonged life, and carefully gloss over the quality of that life. And it's not just inhaler advertisements that perform this sleight-of-hand, but our expectations of nearly every medication or surgery. The latest biological anti-cancer agent promises to extend the average lifespan for metastatic lung cancer from 6 months to 8 months. I am sure that it does do this, on average. "Who wouldn't want another chance?" is the byline. Unfortunately, the drug does not deliver two months of health and energy; it delivers an extra two months of the last few months of life with metastatic cancer. In other words, it delivers two months of pain, constipation, tubes, hospital visits, and side effects. How many would actually choose this if they knew what "another chance" really meant? When polled, very few physicians would actually choose many of these heroic end-of-life type treatments; we know and have seen too much.

"Sometimes I... can't sleep... real well and... just need something."

There is no treatment for Mrs. J____'s anxiety, because it stems from her breath. I can't fix her lungs. Eventually the medications stop working well. Eventually the anxiety wins out and people call the ambulance and are taken to the hospital. There, we routinely hook up a fancy CPAP machine with a mask, and artificially blow air in and out of the lungs, temporarily at least relieving some of the work of breathing. And we try the IV forms of the medications, slightly more powerful, with quicker onset. The patient stays in the hospital a few days until the mask can be removed, and then goes home, praying that the cycle won't start again, which it does of course, inevitably. Sometimes patients have become so weakened in their muscles by constant overuse that the mask with the machine is required; without the blowing pressurized air, the patient simply can no longer breathe on their own. The effort to simply raise and lower the chest is beyond them. And yet, they live on, tied to the "blower", with the mask strapped to the face and the seal around the nose slowly rubbing off the skin as raw red areas appear, and we tighten down the straps holding on the mask as we have to bump up the pressure on the blower. The machine blows air onto the face and down the throat like a 45-mph wind. These patients can't breathe unless they have the equivalent of their head stuck out the window while driving down the highway. No one can tolerate that for very long.

"Mrs. J___, did you talk to your husband about whether you would want to go back to the hospital if your breathing got worse again?" Or sometimes I deliberately phrase this question, "Mrs. J___, did you talk to your husband about whether you will want to go back to the hospital when your breathing gets worse again?" To me the difference in phrasing seems important. For Mrs. J____, it seems to amount to the same thing.

“I told big Jim... but I... have not told little Jim.” She refers to her husband and grandson. “Jimmy, he... he doesn’t like that.”

Jimmy lives with them and takes care of them both. He is dedicated. Shops, transports, and fills the pill dispensers. The younger you are, the less that “giving up” seems to make sense. She told me she doesn’t want the “blower” again, doesn’t want the pokes and lights and the noise of another 5-day hospital stay. But her grandson does want it. The family always wants “to do everything.” How could you not do something if it can prolong your loved one’s life? It seems inhuman almost. A few patients are easily able to tell their families that they are tired, and done with the fight. But most have trouble. They don’t want to let their family down; they are so used to fighting this disease, for years of treatments and x-rays and doctors’ appointments. Most families simply don’t want to talk about it at all. Perhaps it will all just go away if we don’t talk about that now.

Anxiety is not a disease; it is a state of being. In the corner, the oxygen concentrator hums along putting out its two liters per minute of concentrated oxygen, to travel down the flexible tube coiled on the floor, up to the cannula perched on the nose. What can a person do when her master organ is failing? The usual medications we use are "bronchodilators" that are carried down into the lungs with the breath and act on receptors on the smooth muscles in the lungs, relaxing them and opening up the tiny airways, allowing a little more air to pass a little more easily. The medications are given in a nebulizer machine, which simply takes the medication mixed in saline and atomizes it into miniature drops that appears as a cloud of steam and can easily be inhaled through a pipe. The membrane between outside and inside is so thin down in the lungs that inhalation is actually a very effective means of administering drugs. Ironically, the immediate high from dragging on the nicotine in a cigarette is how most patients end up needing the other inhaled medications.

As the master organ founders, there is one other medicine we can use: morphine. Morphine takes away the anxiety of not being able to breathe. Morphine can be swallowed, injected, or even nebulized in steam right into the lungs. In any form it stops someone from caring that they can't breathe. It doesn't cure any disease, it doesn't actually improve the breathing. But no one has to suffocate any longer, gasping and panting, stuck between not wanting further intensive care, but not wanting to pant hideously at home. Morphine, sweet morphine, the source of our scourge of an opioid epidemic, has a wonderful place for those who have run their race, and are ready for comfort.

Calmness means controlling one's breath and with COPD this becomes nearly impossible. Meditation involves focusing on the breath, in and out, with regularity and nothing else in the mind, just the breath, in and out, out and in. I watch Mrs. J___ breathe. I watch her entire body tense up to heave her chest up and back, to open up the lungs and suck air into an already over-expanded space, and then use all the muscles of the chest wall to squeeze, squeeze out the air, back the way it came, up from the lungs through the damaged and soft passages full of mucous, up the throat and out the mouth. I am somehow supposed to counsel this woman on anxiety and separate it out and treat it. As if anxiety were a symptom and not a mode of being itself. I am reminded that gravity is not a separate force of nature, but instead constructs the very fabric of space. Just so, breathing constructs the very fabric of our existence and cannot really be said to cause anxiety, nor to cure it. We live in a universe defined by gravity which is so pervasive we often forget it is there. Our existence is defined by our breath in the same way, and often forgotten by the healthy in the same manner. We can no more forget to breathe than we can forget to be held to earth by gravity. We cannot ask the breathless person to "calm down" any more than we can ask a person to suspend themselves in mid-air. Breath constitutes the fabric of our space-time. When breath fails, so do we.

I Have All the Symptoms of Aging

> *"Love is responsibility of an I for a You: in this consists what cannot consist in any feeling - the equality of all lovers.."* *--Martin Buber, I and Thou*

Portland, also known as "Stumptown" due to its history of large-scale tree felling required to build a city in the middle of a thick woods, remains sparsely forested on the eastside. Yet, from time to time one comes across a small stand of old-growth Douglas fir, towering up and over the puny lawns and clapboard houses beneath. Somehow these woods, the original timber inhabitants of this land, still persist in small stands scattered across the eastside neighborhoods. The giant evergreens, with trunk diameters of twenty feet, were left to guard the clusters of building beneath them.

They are so large that the 3-bedroom ranches and classic Portland Craftsman bungalows appear as if mere toys, scattered on a schoolyard. The Douglas fir is the state tree of Oregon, and with reason, for it looks as if it belongs here. What story lies behind the sparing of these trees when all around the boulevards were clearcut to make way for houses? We dwell beneath these watchers, who watched over the Kwakiut'l and Lewis and Clark, and now us as we attempt to become indigenous.

I arrive at one such sheltered neighborhood on a sunny late afternoon, with the low-angled sun beaming between furrowed brown trunks. My destination is a small house that sits on a small lot with not one, but two, of these giants sprouting up out of the yard. The roots themselves seem to be raising the earth, and the small house will soon be carried away on an arboreal wave.

We sit, as usual, at the table in the dining nook. Francis is my patient, an elderly woman with the usual panoply of chronic illnesses and bottles of pills. She was a nurse, and worked at most of the local hospitals at one point or another in her long career. Like all health professionals, she evinces a biting cynicism about life and the conditions that she once treated but have now caught up with her.

“I guess you might say that I did fall, yes, but it wasn't really a fall... I stumbled.”

"Were you here in the house? In the living room?" I try to get a sense of what she was doing when she "sort of fell." No one wants to admit to falling, to that loss of mastery over one's own body, the body we order around for decades to do our bidding and then suddenly it rebels.

We continue to talk when another woman walks in from the periphery of my vision, and stands, leaning against the kitchen counter. There was no introduction as I entered the house, no acknowledgement of another person there to participate in my visit. Yet, here, coolly observing, stands someone else who clearly lives here, and belongs in this house.

There are categories of people that one lets into one's home. There are service workers who fix dishwashers and electrical cables. And then there are friends and family who are welcomed joyously. When the cable guy shows up, you don't introduce him to your whole family. When a friend arrives it would be impolite not to introduce her. Somewhere in between is your house call doctor, both a service worker and a family intimate, providing a check on how the plumbing is working but also exploring the most intimate depths of life, love and death. So I am not introduced to the other woman standing at the counter as we talk.

"It was hardly anything," Francis continues, and the newcomer grimaces in the background.

"You should know, she has fallen a few times. In fact, about every week," the newcomer finally adds.

Clearly this watcher is not just an observer, but an active member of this household, and I am missing my best chance to find out what is really going on here. "Yes... hi, I'm Dr. Benson, I don't think we met..." I trail off.

"I am Shirley and we're housemates."

"Wonderful, well it sounds like you have seen her be a little unsteady sometimes."

"I don't think I would call it unsteady," Francis breaks in. "Sometimes the dog gets in my way."

There is indeed a dog, an ancient graying spaniel that clearly does not move too frequently from its bed. In the background Shirley rolls her eyes. I change tactics and ask, "So Shirley, you have seen Francis be a little more unsteady lately?"

"Not just lately, she has been falling for a year at least."

I am still trying to place how Shirley knows about Francis's health and situation. "So you are here all the time?"

They both laugh. "We met in 1965 when we were nurses at Providence hospital. We have been housemates ever since."

"So that's... 50 years ago!"

"Oh yes! I know everything about her," Shirley continues, with heavy emphasis on the "everything". "We have adopted a lot of dogs, fifteen I think. Max there is the latest one we got from the shelter. But he doesn't do much, and he is not what she is tripping over."

Francis gives her an angry glance. What really is the relationship between these two old nurses? Shirley is healthy and spry. Francis has heart disease, diabetes and atrial fibrillation. She has suffered numerous small strokes. I ask her to show me how she checks her blood sugars, and as she fumbles with the test strips for the glucometer machine, it becomes clear that she cannot really be checking her blood sugars at all.

"Let's look at your medications," I announce as the clock ticks through the hour I have scheduled here. Francis brings out some pill bottles. Shirley hovers beside the table as we check off each bottle and talk about it.

"Well, the metformin there she stopped taking after the last stroke. The doctor said her kidneys weren't working well enough for it to be safe," Shirley interjects.

"No, that's not what he said," counters Francis. "I just don't take them as often now. I take them just once a day."

The bottle states, "Take twice daily," but is dated from six months ago, prior to the last hospitalization. Any combination of what these two have said could be the correct interpretation of various doctors' advice. Metformin is an excellent medication for diabetes because it reduces the body's resistance to its own natural insulin. The patient can take less insulin, or use fewer drugs that stimulate more insulin production, and thereby control blood sugars without weight gain. But when the kidneys are not working well, metformin is more likely to cause the side-effect of bypassing the usual metabolic pathway for energy production and so cause a dangerous buildup of lactic acid in the body, lactic acidosis. As the various organ systems slowly fail with long-standing diabetes, or simply long-standing aging, each medication becomes less and less useful. The inevitable side-effects that any drug has start to outweigh its possible benefits. Hypertension medications prevent heart attack and stroke, but eventually the lowered blood pressure in the brain just causes dizziness and lightheadedness. Chemotherapy agents control cancer growth, but as the body weakens or the cancer metastasizes, they simply cause nausea, vomiting and weakness without actually helping the patient. Wisdom consists in knowing when the medications are helping, and then gracefully abandoning them as they start to do more harm than good.

Francis easily becomes confused regarding her health and pill bottles. She covers for this confusion by joking. She has a sense of humor about her body's failings and weaknesses. Yet this is a fully competent nurse who once took care of complex patients in the hospital. She is, or was, capable of understanding her health conditions, and much more. Likely the confusion reflects some degree of dementia. The combination of diabetes and history of strokes means this dementia may be what is called "vascular dementia". Unlike Alzheimers, where the underlying brain mechanism remains unknown, vascular dementia stems from numerous small strokes killing tiny areas of brain tissue. Over time, the microscopic areas of dead neurons accumulate and minor errors in thinking multiply into full memory loss and confusion. Unlike Alzheimers, where we at least have a few medications that can prolong brain functioning for a short time, in vascular dementia there is simply no treatment. Of course, we use medications like blood thinners to try to prevent future strokes, but the strokes in this disease come from chronically damaged walls in microscopic arteries, the arterioles, rather than large blood clots flicking off from the heart or carotid arteries. In other words, the damage has been done by 20 years of diabetes, and no medication can go back in time.

Shirley has been propping up Francis's failing faculties for some time now, silently, or not so silently, nudging and cajoling from the background. How in the world did these two old nurses end up meeting and then becoming housemates for 40 years? Doctors are supposed to probe and take a "social history", which includes what we euphemistically call the "social determinants of disease".

Usually this amounts to asking about smoking and alcohol consumption, and occasionally ventures out to marital status, presumably because this reflects whether there is family support at home. These questions are part of the required elements for billing codes, and insurance companies have determined that they are necessary to meet the highest code status for maximum reimbursement. Without such a mandate would we even make these perfunctory inquiries?

For chronic diseases, the social determinants of disease are the whole ball of wax. It is the whole story, and it would take an entire book to relate a person's life in a form that does justice to an adequate explanation of how that life impacts physical health. The old school family doctor used to know their patients to the level of a novel per person. Now, with 10-minute visits, the doctor, struggling to manhandle the electronic record, gets by with "Do you smoke?" Many bright students choose medicine as a profession after getting excited about proteins in the lab. Eventually they realize that test tubes are fine, but they want to read the book of life. More and more, providers are burned out and fleeing medicine because the book of life they found was a billing and coding manual.

How much should I probe into Francis and Shirley's relationship and home life? Back in the 1960's, the options for publicly declaring an "alternative" lifestyle were culturally limited and perhaps dangerous. I had a great-aunt who was my most devoted "Auntie" growing up, travelling twice yearly to see us, bringing presents and bringing love. She had gotten married, and then left the man two days later and spent the rest of her life with her "friend", Mrs. Combs. No one ever spoke about that relationship or what it portended. As a child, my great-aunt was simply the most loving person in my life. Now, in Portland at least, few seem to care who you live with or what you do in your house. There exists a whole medical literature of gay and lesbian health, but it doesn't address how to deal with vascular dementia and diabetes care. Does it matter how these two met or the specifics of how they interacted in the past? Perhaps eventually it might, but on my first visit here under these old-growth trees would such questions build our relationship or undermine it? Physicians are encouraged to probe into sexuality, even in the elderly. But these exhortations are always couched in the language of the social determinants of disease where sexuality is certainly important. There is another level to the provider-patient relationship, that of building trust and cultivating an emotional storehouse to draw on in the future.

I almost ask about those early days 40 years ago, hesitate and then stop. I want to know what it would have been like, rebelling against the cultural expectation of marriage and family. I want to know how they built up a partnership that has lasted until now, with Shirley now standing in for Francis's missing brain cells. But I wait and don't ask. Not yet. These Douglas fir have been here for a long time, growing slowly. There is no rush, they teach me. Whatever brought these two together will last until the next time I am here. The roots are strong and deep and the crown touches the sky.

Yes, I Am a Complex Patient

"In medicine, too, we are trying to deliver a range of services to millions of people at a reasonable cost and with a consistent level of quality. Unlike the Cheesecake Factory, we haven't figured out how." -- *Atul Gawande, Big Med*

A month has passed, and I am back up the hill checking on Michael. He walks to the door to greet me this time, rather than just staying seated at his table. The sun is shining today, and it illuminates a field stretching out from the window, green to infinity. There had been a lot of work behind the scenes since the last time I was here. Of course, he cancelled the sleep clinic appointment. Why? The timing wasn't right, or there was a grand-niece visiting, or a hundred other real-life events intervened. Sitting behind the desk at a hospital, clinic, or other healthcare facility, it appears that the world revolves around your schedule and your institution. From the living room, it is so clear how wrong that assumption is. It turns out people are not usually sitting around counting the hours until their doctor's appointment. They are not thinking, I need this so I can go on with my life. Their life goes on and sometimes they fit medical care into it. And so we helped Michael reschedule the sleep visit. In fact, we helped reschedule it three times. Despite explanations and harangues, Michael did not intuitively see why this was so important. He had not studied the physiologic pathways that create heart failure from disordered breathing, and the gurgling breathless death that heart failure can conjure. He had not seen these effects first-hand. He just had the patient education sheet which dryly lists causes and effects, like a restaurant menu. So we kept reaching out to him rather than just waiting for him to ask for help.

He finally did go and see the sleep doctor who repeated what I had told him: it is really really important to sleep correctly. Then the actual CPAP device, the small box that has a motor that concentrates the air and blows it down a tube, into a mask, and finally down the patient's airways, forcing open the throat and lungs, was not delivered. Our nursing team spent hours sleuthing out which company was supposed to deliver it, when it would be delivered with the respiratory therapist to set it up.

I thought Michael looked good, but I couldn't tell why. "It's because I trimmed down my beard doc," he finally said. "The mask wasn't sealing around my thick mustache, so they made me trim it." And perhaps the bags under his eyes are less swollen and thick.

"You have been sleeping!" I exclaim.

"Some," he replies, "I have the machine and I get on it for a few hours. I spend a few hours in bed on the CPAP. Sometimes I awaken about 2 or 3 and come out here. And then I might nap in the chair a little bit."

After Michael's forceful resistance to this routine, the actual use of the CPAP seems like a minor miracle. No wonder he looks like he has rested.
"He's not telling you, but he has lost some weight too," his wife adds excitedly.

He gives her a withering look and admits his blood sugar levels have been lower. "Sometimes I wake up and feel just... weird," he adds. "I usually get some orange juice."

I never imagined his sugars would improve this fast with the CPAP and I start to worry. Low blood sugar, or hypoglycemia, is much more dangerous than high blood sugars. Classically the health care world has focused on the high blood sugars that define diabetes as a condition, and over the long-run it is true that high sugars are destructive to every organ. But in the short run, you can die from low blood sugar. The brain particularly is susceptible to low blood sugar levels, and episodes without enough brain food are like mini-strokes, depriving neurons of their fuel and actually killing them off. People who end up with very main low blood sugar episodes perform worse on cognitive tests, they get dementia, they get a brain fog.

"Have you tested your blood sugars when you feel odd?" I enquire.

"Yes, and the lowest I have seen is 100 on the meter." This is a little reassuring, but only a little. The glucometer meters are not completely accurate, and the blood sugar level measured by a finger-prick can be quite different from the levels circulating in the main arteries and up to the brain. We need to decrease Michael's insulin immediately. The use of the CPAP has indeed decreased his adrenaline surges and thereby his sugar levels. Now, we can use less insulin and accelerate his weight loss.

"I often wake up at night with tingling in my arms." This is new since starting the CPAP, and puzzling. It takes 10 minutes of clarification to discover that the tingling happens only at night while on the CPAP, is affected by the position of his body while sleeping, and goes away once he is up walking around again. It appears that he has some mild arm swelling that occurs while on the breathing machine, and the extra fluid in his arms causes mild nerve compression which causes tingling. What could cause this unusual effect? Could his heart's pumping be affected enough to change his water retention? Insulin, being a large molecule, also attracts water through its osmotic effect, and causes some fluid retention; Michael does use a whopping dose of insulin. I cut his insulin dose in half and arrange some follow up nursing calls every day for a little while, to check on his sugars and odd swelling symptoms.

In many ways, Michael seems like he hardly needs our concierge home-care service. He is independent, mobile, and wealthy. Yet, despite all that his health was deteriorating rapidly due to a confusing mess of diseases and treatments culminating in a severe mistrust of the medical system and its ability to actually help him. He had heard so many specialists' advice regarding his health, and been unable to implement any of it, and had seen no improvement in his condition, that he had given up on the whole endeavor. I like to think that his other doctors had told him much the same things that I had: diet, the utility of the CPAP machine, exercise, all the good things that we get paid to lecture others about. The difference was that I had sat in his house for an hour to start with, and listened to him, and not discounted his troubles. I had listened to the whole story, the whole bucket of frustrations stemming from 15 years of skewed interactions, the vehemence of his irritation.

Doctors are trained now to establish the expectation with patients that they will handle one thing in a visit. The front staff in a clinic will state this while scheduling the visit weeks ahead of time, "Have your issue chosen so the doctor can get right to it." Most clinic visits are 15 minutes maximum, and that is the doctor's time, not face-to-face time with the patient, which is usually only 5-10 minutes. In that type of encounter, there is only time for one complaint, with a few questions, a review of medications, a cursory exam, and then a "solution." The solution is nearly always "correct", in the sense that if implemented it would improve the patient's life. And if you just have one problem when you walk in the door, like a sore throat, the solution will help you: gargle some salt water, or take this antibiotic for strep throat, or whatever. But when the one problem is enmeshed in a panoply of others, which are all tied up in a lifestyle and habits not easily changed by a line of advice, then the clinic visit becomes nearly useless.

Unlike most of my patients, Michael actually has resources. He owns an RV and when he feels better his goal is to take a trip. He was a successful business owner and able to make calculated decisions weighing evidence. And yet, he could not make the healthcare system work for him and was slowly dying of preventable diseases.

People who have straight-forward health issues appear to be able to make rational health decisions and manage their own care. They might consider their health needs, evaluate the insurance plans available to them, and make a reasonable decision as to the best plan. They might also evaluate their doctors and treatments and costs, just as a good businessman might. Somewhere, however as a person accumulates complex diseases, the ability to make reasonable decisions and then act on them in the healthcare realm disappears under a mountain of evidence. Most primary care doctors can't even keep up with the complexity of a patient like Michael. They can't sort out how to juggle the interacting physiological pieces, and drugs, and procedures. They can't effectively intervene to improve these people's lives. How then can the patients themselves make rational decisions? And yet, without the assumption of rational decisions, the premise behind a health care "market" collapses in a heap of pills, procedures and paperwork. We might be able to rationally choose where to go to have an MRI done based on the price and how convenient the hours are. But no one can rationally choose how best to tackle 6 chronic conditions that have complex interactions amongst each other and with various social determinants such as location, access, race, gender and a hundred others. There is no assembly line that will turn out perfectly healthy humans. It's a mess out there.

Violence Here is a Social Norm

"Sing, O goddess, the anger of Achilles son of Peleus, that brought countless ills upon the Achaeans. Many a brave soul did it send hurrying down to Hades."
--Homer, The Iliad

I have come to appreciate the finer points of trailer homes. Most of my patients live in mobile homes. There is perhaps something profound in this observation. Mobile homes around Portland cost about $100,000. The median home price in Portland is now $416,000. Most of my patients purchased their mobile homes back when the price was little more than the cost of a car. Today, I am in the home of a 90-year-old who sits in his ubiquitous recliner, clutching a bottle of whiskey in his right hand.

"I feel comfortable with the bottle. I just like to sip it."

The heart failure, the lung disease, the swollen legs propped on pillows are all familiar to me. But conducting a medical visit while my patient sips whiskey is new. Occasionally even the most jaded can be surprised.

The mobile home is comfortable. "Lived-in" would be the most appropriate word. Mobile homes are built from lighter -- and cheaper -- materials, and they have a certain patina they acquire as they age long past the planned time of obsolescence. A classic old Portland Craftsman will have an aged oak musty smell. An aging mobile home smells instead like a motel. Solid wood rounds out beautifully under a hundred years of footfalls and sliding hands. Particle board warps and crumbles instead. It is easy to feel dignified on a leather sofa in a polished Craftsman. From a threadbare chair next to a metal window, dignity requires more effort, but is no less attainable, and perhaps more precious due to being harder won. It is only 10am, and the tightly clasped whiskey bottle portends a complex tale.

"You live here with your wife and son?" I ask.

"They say he is my 'son'," he retorts, "but I don't think so."

"Ohh... but he does live here?" I cautiously probe into a dynamic that could lead anywhere, including into the social quicksand.

"Damn him, he lives here all right. Let me show you what he called me last night. You wouldn't believe how he was swearing." Mr. T pulls out a rumpled scrap of paper where he has carefully block printed a list of swear words.

"He called you all these things last night?" A vision of a whiskey-fueled yelling match appears before me, replete with slamming screen doors and "Stella! Stella!" ringing out into the night. Except that Mr. T is 90 years old and requires a walker to get around his house.

"Well, I won't take that kind of thing from him," he went on. "I slammed him up against the wall back there in the hall. I told him to apologize."

If this sort of thing was actually taking place I would be required to report it to Adult Protective Services. Healthcare workers are "mandatory reporters" of any potential abuse at any age. But this feeble old man seemed unlikely to be slamming anything up against the flimsy wall of his manufactured home.

"When did that happen? That sounds rough," I open up the conversation for him to share more about it.

"Yes, last night," he continues, eager to talk about it. "That good-for-nothing wouldn't shut up, I gave him the what-for!"

"What were you drinking last night?"
"I had my usual, beer in the evening. I like to sip on the whiskey during the day because the beer gets warm. At night I prefer beer."

"How much can you drink in an evening?"

"I have a case in the fridge and I can mostly get through that," he recounts almost proudly. "I learned to drink pretty young. My daddy drank and then I did too. I just missed the war, too young," he continued. "And afterwards the military was laying off people so I joined the police. I was a cop my whole life. I learned how to take someone down so they don't give you no trouble."

I have to do some mental arithmetic to be sure I am thinking about the right "war" when he tosses off this phrase. So many patients, so many wars they have been in. At age 90 he would have been just too young for World War II.

"Hey doctor," I hear from the back room. Mr. T's daughter is in the back room and calls to me to come over. I excuse myself and walk to the back of the trailer.

"None of that happened," she says worriedly, "he cusses some but I don't want you to think it's like that around here."

"How does he get the booze if he can't even get out of the house?" I ask.

"His wife buys it. She shouldn't. She's not my mother, but we get on fine," she adds when she sees my quizzical look. I return to Mr. T and ask him more about his life before retirement.

"I won the sharpshooting prize three years straight. I could toss up a can, and before it even fell, draw and shoot it clean through. No one could shoot like me. I gave up my guns though, I don't have any now. On account of my temper. My wife said it would be best."

I am inclined to agree with her assessment.

"See that case over there," he points to the shelves below the television, "that's a Civil War bullet, a real one. I just have the best pieces of my collection now. No room for all of it."

He likes to talk, and will tell me stories indefinitely. "See my left hand here? I can't really move the finger. It didn't heal right after I got in a fight outside the bar back in '67. The other guy got the worst of it though. I hit him real good! We could get in trouble, fighting off-duty like that. So I ran, and never had it looked at by the doctor. I know there's nothing you can do about it now. It doesn't stop me from holding this bottle though," he gives a little laugh.

Mr. T has my patients' usual suite of diseases, and the swollen legs with a small non-healing wound. He appears to get most of his "nutrition" from alcohol, which actually has a lot of calories, to most drinkers' surprise. But of course these calories are empty of protein, and so contribute to the low level of protein in his blood, protein that keeps the fluid in the arteries and veins through osmotic pressure. So fluid leaks, his body and his legs swell. Wounds develop and never heal because there is none of the protein or vitamins that are needed to form new tissue. The pathophysiology is as old as the invention of alcohol, and as familiar to healthcare as the gunshot wound. The biochemical pathways are learned and re-learned through medical training until they become instinct. They can seem challenging to pre-medical students trying to cram for an entrance exam, but for the practicing clinician, they are second nature. Been there, done that. Boring.

Many years ago I staffed an emergency room in a small town and became an expert in treating the ravages of alcohol: swollen legs, liver failure with jaundiced eyes and bulging bellies, bleeding ulcers and esophageal varices. When enough liver cells are destroyed by alcohol, the circulation from the intestines through the liver backs up and extra fluid appears in the abdomen. Called ascites, this clear yellowish fluid can build up in huge quantities, swelling the abdomen and causing pain, sometimes even massive infection as gut contents leak out into the normally sterile area. Many doctors become experts in tapping the abdominal cavity to drain this fluid. The procedure is strangely satisfying, swabbing the protuberant abdominal wall with betadine, numbing it with lidocaine and then jabbing a long needle straight in, and watching while liters of this urine-like fluid flows out through the tube into jar after jar after jar. The abdominal pressure is relieved, at least for a few days or weeks, and I bundle them home from the emergency room, washing my hands with satisfaction.

After twenty years the procedure remains the same, but the meaning behind it has changed. In fact, it has lost its meaning. It has become just a series of hand movements, of manual skills. The meaning lay in the challenge, and now the challenge is gone. How do we find meaning in our everyday activities? My remarkable conclusion after years of practice is that there is nothing inherent in the doctor's task that creates meaning. We find meaning only because something resonates. And reverberation requires a chamber, a container that already exists. How do I make sense of this tragic family existing on the edge of sanity on the edge of Portland? Are they just another "can you believe it" story to swap at some future medical conference?

I took a Hippocratic oath which said something about helping other people, and my ability to make any inroads in this multi-generational tragedy appears minimal. The meaning in my encounter with them does not lie in the biochemical pathways I can affect by manipulating drugs and lifestyle and drinking. The meaning arises from something more fundamentally human, the stories that can make sense of triumph or tragedy. Because I have heard other stories, do these stories strike me in a different way? I argue for humanism in medicine, but what does that really mean? Does it mean that I have "heard it all before"? Every doctor has heard it all before on some level. We all experience enough raw life in our training that nothing is really a surprise anymore: not the vibrators retrieved from rectal cavities, not the gruesome fungating cancer eating away a breast, not the shocked family who just learned their child has leukemia. But it's not just the callous approach from having seen humans *in extremis* that constitutes humanism in medicine. Humanism means placing extreme stories into a larger context. The cycle of poverty and violence makes sense when one has read the Greek cycle of Agamemnon, cursed by his father's murder of his brother's twins. Having "seen it all" predisposes to a burned-out cynicism in healthcare providers. But taking "seen it all" and morphing that into "I have personally experienced the truth of great literature" instead creates a resilience and a perspective that allows transcendence of the impossible black holes we encounter in the world.

The humanistic perspective saves doctors, but does it also help patients? I do know that after hundreds of stories of alcoholism leading to destruction, the cynical self-preserving doctor usually just goes through the motions of providing good care. And the motions of care do not constitute actual good care. The cynical glaze of the overworked doctor can be pierced by a larger perspective and allow providers to continue to feel, to continue to experience tragedy, rather than walling it off for survival. We need a vehicle to carry us through the wall of routine bureaucracy so we can always come back to the real humans that we encounter. The immediate need of the person sitting in front of us often hides the experience of that need; the immediacy of the patient hides the person behind the patient. Humanism pierces that veil.

Mr. T grew up in violence, saw his life's work through the prism of violence, and now in his waning days only knows how to make sense of his life by telling stories about violence. Medicine has been tasked with tackling nearly all of society's woes in the modern era. I am likely the last connection Mr. T has to the wider culture and its resources. Every modern society spends about the same amount on the combination of medical care and social services. For whatever reason, America has decided to put all of that money into medicine and very little into other social services. So I am the tip of the medical spear, thrust through the creaking screen door, poking away at bandages and bullets. Violent exploits give this life meaning and I will have to enter that world to even get started.

My education on violence began in my first semester of college, my very first lecture as an undergraduate. We had been assigned to read the Iliad over the summer prior to arriving at Reed College. I read it; I understood nothing. Why are there hundreds of pages describing gangs of barbarians slaughtering each other? This is great literature? I filed into the lecture hall early Monday morning, ready with my notepad, trying to look academic. I recall forgetting to take notes as I sat mesmerized by a lecture on how the Iliad functioned as a foundational poem for Greek civilization, recounting the woes that humans create through overweening pride, anger, and sometimes the sheer fate of the gods. The Iliad, the shared account of the Bronze-Age barbarism humans were emerging from as Greek civilization flourished, constituted the beginnings of humanism. I learned that day that we read about Achilles because his story reflects something fundamental about being human. We are all but a moment of pride away from sinking back into barbarism, and the Iliad will not let you forget this brutal fact. Humanism prevents doctors from collapsing the person down into their chemistry, and worse, collapsing everyone's chemistries into a generic routine. Stories make us human, and without them it's just one damn thing after the next.

The Manhattan Project

"Beautiful! Great God! His yellow skin scarcely covered the work of muscles and arteries beneath; his hair was of a lustrous black, and flowing; but these luxuriances only formed a more horrid contrast with his watery eyes, that seemed almost of the same colour as the dun-white sockets in which they were set, his shrivelled complexion and straight black lips."
-- Mary Shelley, Frankenstein or the modern Prometheus

Mr. Kraemer moved to this adult foster care home three weeks ago. Foster care homes are a remarkable new advancement in senior living where private individuals can relatively easily take on elderly boarders in their homes. Rather than requiring the expense of "nursing homes," people can live in a small community of 5-6, in a nearly home-like environment. The caregivers make a living, the residents get a non-institutional life, and families can keep their aging relatives nearby. Mr Kraemer of course wished that he was still in his own private home.

"Just last year we were still going out in the boat and fishing," his daughter Betty explains. "He just let his legs go I guess. Then he fell. Twice. His house was a mess and it just wasn't safe." She is in tears now.

I can see from the door that Mr. Kraemer's legs indeed are a mess. They are enormous, swollen and weeping fluid, saturating the wraps that struggle to contain bulging flesh and fluid. Dementia has sapped away a lot of awareness of his current situation, but he remembers a lot of the past.

"We built our house out around here. It was open back then, fields and trees." He looks around wildly, encountering just the flat walls of his small room. He is, of course, not living in his own house now. Three weeks ago he moved in here to the foster home. I wonder if we could have helped keep him in his own home longer if we had been called in sooner. Still, this is a great spot, with excellent care. The caregiver is willing to change his leg dressings daily, and not many will do so.

The skin is stretched tight like a water balloon, but a balloon that leaks. The medicine list with its 15 entries does not seem to be helping this problem much. There are medications for every organ system in the human body. Eye drops for glaucoma, inhalers for emphysema, combination pills for the heart-kidney hormonal interactions, bladder anti-spasmodics to combat the load of urine the kidneys produce from the diuretics, and even topical skin powders to prevent yeast growing in moist skin folds. It can be difficult to ferret out how and when and why these medicines got started. No one starts 15 at once of course. To accumulate this many requires the work of years and hundreds of doctors and hospital stays.

Each medication arrives with a package insert detailing in small print all the manufacturing that has gone into creating that particular molecule and its various fillers packaged into a tablet. No one spends much time with these inserts and they are included simply because that is the law; pharmaceuticals are required to supply this information. First, the drug molecule starts as a potential drug, screened in panels of thousands of similar molecules. Then when it shows potential, the drug is tested extensively in animals for safety. Finally the drug has a few limited human trials before undergoing a large study with hundreds of patients. After receiving an approval from the government agencies, it is finally mass produced and marketed in medical journals and increasingly on television. The resources to create even one useful molecule are breathtaking and a true testament to human scientific achievement. Mr. Kraemer takes 15 of these molecules, and has been tried on another 20 that were ultimately deemed not useful for him. We stand on the shoulders of giants indeed. It seems that the 315 pounds of man wedged into a recliner might be better seen as balancing precariously on a pinnacle of achievement.

The peculiar aspect of package inserts with complex patients like Mr. Kraemer is that none of his medications have ever been tested all together in one body. The exact combination of 15 molecules that are used in this particular Homo sapiens have likely never been seen before. Does it matter? Perhaps not. We have some knowledge of what the interactions between the chemicals might be, and what the interactions with the body's own systems might be. And yet, the subtle combinations might matter; they might even matter a lot. The problem is that we do not know, and likely have no way of ever knowing because the scientific method requires controlling for unknown factors and only testing the intervention we want to understand. We will never find another patient like Mr. Kraemer and can never "control" for all the factors affecting his health and outcome. There will never be a randomized trial of 93-year-olds taking all 15 of these medications at once, looking to see whether adding a sixteenth would benefit.

The swelling, or edema, in these legs came on gradually and likely has a combination of causes. There are some obvious contributors, like heart failure causing the heart to not pump as strongly, which then causes the kidneys to not receive as much circulating blood, which makes them secrete hormones to retain fluid to compensate and try to increase the circulating blood volume. When our ancient ancestors were bleeding from a wound, this hormonal mechanism was likely adaptive for survival, by conserving fluid so that we did not die from shock. But now in Mr. Kraemer this feedback mechanism is causing him to retain too much fluid, and swells his legs.

Additionally, the veins in Mr. Kraemer's legs likely are not functioning well. The miniature valves inside the legs are blown out, causing blood to flow back down the legs instead of being supported at each stage back up to the heart by small valves every few inches in healthy veins. A sedentary life contributes to this effect by the resulting lack of pressure from muscle contractions in the calves and thighs to squeeze the blood back up to the abdomen.

So, over time, doctors have compensated by adding heart-failure medicines to squeeze a little more out of each contraction of the heart, and diuretics to squeeze a little more out of the kidneys as they filter the blood. And now, in the last few months, the doctors have acknowledged defeat with their armamentarium of potions and sent Mr. Kraemer to the wound care clinic to have compression wrappings placed on his legs twice a week. There is nothing like physical exterior pressure from a tight wrapping on the skin to combat the interior pressure of blood and fluid under the skin. Twice weekly he gets out of his recliner, transfers awkwardly into a waiting wheelchair, wheels down the ramp and into a waiting medical transport van. He exits at the wound clinic, sits waiting in the waiting room before finally having the old wraps cut off by an expert nurse, greeting the attending physician briefly who checks the weeping wounds, before being packaged up again with fresh clean white gauze and heading back home four hours later. The wound care clinic has hundreds of these patients daily, a virtual factory of soaked gauze and stained elastic wraps.

"We pay $500 a week to transport him to the clinic," Betty explains to me. Of course, Mr. Kraemer also gets transport to his primary care office, and his cardiologist and his nephrologist periodically. I look back and see that each provider has tweaked some medications to attempt to keep the delicate balance of this fragile body.

The television plays sports today as we sit and talk in his small room. More often than not sports are playing when I visit patients. There is a strange irony in watching athletes with near-perfect flawless bodies perform strenuous maneuvers while we tend to bodies on the opposite end of the performance spectrum. The room has been decorated with photos from Mr. Kraemer's past. There is the wedding photo in its false 1950's color of a young couple. Model tractors cover the shelves. Ask about any model of tractor ever produced and Mr. Kraemer can still wax poetic about its horsepower and place of manufacture. He knows tractors even if he doesn't seem to care much about his medicine list.

I glance over across the room to the bed. The sheets are neatly pressed. Too neatly pressed. "How are you sleeping these days, Mr. Kraemer?" I ask with suspicion.

"Fine, just great." he answers.

"But is it hard to get into bed?" I continue.

"Oh yes, too hard. I sleep here in the recliner."

"And you put up your legs with the footrest?" I ask with sinking heart.

"No! It's too uncomfortable, I feel cramped with those. I'm just not flexible like I used to be."

"He doesn't like to get out of his chair," his caregiver Betty chimes in. I look up, way up, from where I am leaned over to the ground tending to his feet. Gravity is a universal force that no one has ever beaten. All of our drug molecules will not beat gravity. And all of our wound care trips will not cheat gravity's inevitable slow push downwards from the abdomen to whatever dangles below it. Humans are designed to vary in position from time to time: sit, walk, even jump and run. I lean back and take a breath as the futility of our healthcare system sinks in.

The cardiologist titrating diuretics never realized that this man never left his recliner with his feet dangling in front of him. The wound care clinic diligently changed his compression bandages twice a week, never knowing that no mere piece of elastic would stop the Newton's law from exerting its force 24 hours a day. The primary care physician, breezing through an office visit with the man in the wheelchair had no idea how he spent his time at home.

Saving Mr. Kraemer's life from his various disease required all the knowledge of innumerable drug package inserts. But the saved life has taken on its own existence, independent of the intricate thought that created it. Swollen limbs, clogged arteries and ratty lungs assembled together form a grotesque creature that we created, and then turn loose into an uncaring world to fend for itself. Was the error the use of science to save body parts? Or was it to abandon these chronically ill bodies to fare for themselves in a world more suited to Olympic athletes?

Nothing in my medical armamentarium can save Mr. Kraemer except the conversation at the foot of the bed. There are no better pills, or robot-assisted surgeries, that will more cunningly attach together these body parts. Only the human conversation at the foot of the chair can unearth the truth behind why Mr. Kraemer never gets better. There is a pattern here. Science keeps creating tools that have complex consequences. The medical tools that keep us alive create unforeseen situations that science itself cannot explain, nor contain.

Examples of scientific advances creating unintended consequences which require humanistic solutions are nearly everywhere today: the atom bomb, genetic cloning, the internet and Facebook, the internal combustion engine and global warming. Nearly every technological advance creates a human mess which human complexivists have to manage. Just like Victor Frankenstein in the novel so long ago, our eagerness for technical solutions outstrips our capacity for caring. Everywhere medicine has built Frankenstein's monsters out of all of us, heedlessly saving our lives over and over by grafting on cunningly crafted solutions to prop up failing body parts. And is not the project a noble one? Who would decline a prolonged life, regardless of the cost? Was Frankenstein's error the creation of the monster or its abandonment? We have created ourselves and now we must bind up the raw edges. So, I gather up the saturated wraps from the floor and start talking about gravity and how to deal with it.

Doctor Heal Thyself

"Medice, cura te ipsum." -- *Luke 4:23*

Beginning doctors don't like this job doing home visits. Medical schools have to concentrate on teaching people to treat diseases. Years of science training produces providers who know how to use scientific tools. What a disaster if they did not. Our modern world has slipped into a miasma of internet conspiracies fueled by uncritical acceptance of theories and suppositions. A science education cannot be replaced as the cornerstone for real medical care. But it does tend to spit out clones who pursue what they know, which is diseases. So, we find diseases everywhere, sometimes losing track of the people we are sworn to treat.

After a rigorous scientific education followed by rigorous clinical training, young people tend to want to find these diseases they have studied for so long. After my residency, I wanted to use my entire training and see and treat every kind of patient. I took a job in rural Wyoming, working at a small hospital where I awoke early, went to the hospital and saw patients there for an hour, then walked down the hall to my clinic where I saw a patient every 15 minutes all day, often going back to the hospital at lunch or after clinic. I also delivered babies and could be interrupted at any moment by my pager with someone in labor. On the weekends, I covered the emergency department, treating everything from coughs to the crushed chest from an ATV rollover. I sewed up the ligaments in a hand torn nearly in half by a grain auger. I was in heaven. We want to use these skills we have spent ten years painfully learning.

Medical education provides a guided mentorship, so after finally graduating, the first patient seen all alone, without any backup, feels like a revelation. And it should, because it takes another few years of independent practice before all the theoretical education consolidates into a comfort with the human condition in its most common physiologic misadventures. But the comfort level does arrive, and most diseases become more routine. The astute clinician comes to understand what should be obvious, what can be cured, what is an ominous sign, and when the end is near. When the science behind the medicine finally becomes intuitive, then another door opens and allows the doctor to glimpse again the true human behind the disease.

This moment happened for me at the same time as my son Noah started to have seizures. He was four years old and wrestling with his two year old brother Ephraim on the carpet of the living room. Ephraim came running because Noah wasn't trying to push him off anymore, which he should have been because he was the bigger, older brother. Except he wasn't really much bigger than his younger brother, because Noah had never developed quite according to the guidelines, always below the 5th percentile, never eating well, vomiting frequently for no apparent reason. Noah seized, and within months he was seizing all the time, daily. Then in a year he was seizing multiple times in a day, and we became frantic parents of illness, not just a family, and not just a self-assured doctor.

Fifteen years later Noah has run through all the tests, all the drugs and all the diets. My wife has devoted her life to caring for him because he never stopped seizing. He still seizes daily. He no longer can speak and requires full time care to eat, and bathe and walk. He is the quintessential frail patient, requiring constant attention to keep him from decompensating and ending up in the hospital.

Noah ties us to the place in ways that few others experience. It is really desperately difficult to take Noah out on trips. First, we get him into the car. Which involves assisting him to walk out there, and then lifting him into this seat. He slumps over, so we have systems to keep him upright. Then we drive, and Noah gets carsick and vomits. Not every time, but enough that we are always wondering if it will happen. So we schedule his meals around the time of the trip, to avoid a full stomach. Eventually we arrive at some destination. Can Noah walk at that point, or will he go in his wheelchair? Because he is out and about, will he miss a meal? He is already so skinny and has such trouble with food intolerances, seizures causing vomiting, and coughing on textures, that keeping him fed is a stressful priority. Finally we arrive at a destination, usually some public place, perhaps even a doctor's office. Then he can seize. For the uninitiated a seizure is a traumatic event, the shaking, the gasping, the frequent vomiting, soiled trousers, the laying down on his side in the first aid "rescue position" so he can breathe. A seizure reminds its witnesses of the human illusion of self-control, that our minds are the masters of our bodies, rather than the reality, which is that usually it is the other way around.

We stay home a lot. Noah likes his home. We can walk around the yard. When the sun is out, we can sit on the bench on the patio. When he was younger, we sent Noah to school for a while, trying to give him a "normal" life. He was in a mainstream classroom and had his own aide. The kids grew to like Noah in their class. He never added anything in particular, silently observing from the corner, sitting by his aide, occasionally flapping a hand excitedly, or more infrequently even having a seizure. Yet Noah looks at people with a piercing gaze that makes you feel good. He looks and looks and looks, following you with his eyes. He doesn't speak but his eyes seem to say something. So the kids often picked him to be on their team for the spelling bee, or bingo. Then he would sit with that team while they played, quietly watching. He accepts anyone and everyone, which is why they liked him so much.

Noah drools, and keeping him looking presentable so not too many people stare is a constant task. He usually wears a bandana, Western style, around his neck to catch the secretions. It becomes saturated and we change it. We have a cupboard full of different colored and patterned bandanas. Noah was distinctive at that small school for a lot of reasons, being the only tiny kid in a wheelchair sleeping in the nurse's office after a seizure. But mostly he looked distinctive because of his blue or red bandanas. We even had one with a pirate print. In the spring, the day arrived for the class photo. Every one of those kids showed up wearing a matching bandana that day. He got his picture taken with his adopted class.

It was clear that Noah brought a gift to his classmates through presence, as he does with everyone. But for Noah, being at school around other little kids just brought exposure to viruses. And with viruses came fevers and uncontrolled non-stop seizures. He was absent more days than he was present, and we eventually retreated back to our home with Noah, where he can be king of his own castle. My two other children grew up with a disabled brother and it is hard to underestimate the impact that has had on them. They are compassionate. They treasure each moment. They have learned something that not everyone gets a chance to see in life.

Noah has suffered through years of his illness and disability. But he does not cry. And in fact he seems strangely content. It's not just because he can't speak that he doesn't complain. He truly is simply living and has no use for complaint. He breathes, or looks around at his family, and that is enough. He eats and watches his favorite show, and that is enough. In fact, everything is just enough for him. Everyone has their motivations for getting up every day, and Noah is mine.

Tso'-lo: Wandering

"Still round the corner there may wait
A new road or a secret gate
And though I oft have passed them by
A day will come at last when I
Shall take the hidden paths that run
West of the Moon, East of the Sun."
-- JRR Tolkien, Lord of the Rings

I have been learning about the Chinook jargon that was spoken here at the mouth of the Columbia for nearly 100 years, from before Lewis and Clark, to 1900. It evolved to allow communication between Chinook and Nootka natives, French trappers and American settlers. It contains a glorious mish-mash of 400 words from all four languages. Tso'-lo is my favorite word, meaning wandering or the wanderer. If history had worked out differently, we might all still be speaking Chinook jargon here on the Columbia, we might still have a creative meeting of equal cultures rather than the destruction which actually occurred. We might learn something about living on the Columbia if we spoke Chinook jargon; it belongs to this place.

My patient today is Barbara. I was consulted to go see her because she could not make it to the clinic anymore. Pulling up at her run-down house I could smell the cigarette smoke wafting out the screen door. There is no car in the driveway. The front step has a wheelchair ramp with an old barbecue at the top, converted from roasting meats to smoldering tobacco long ago, it now performs its function as an ashtray marvelously, overflowing with butts. Barbara has lived here a long time. Long enough that her daughter, who functions as her caregiver, and is the actual chain smoker of the place, has also lived here a long time. Her primary care physician asked me to see her because she has a broken right leg, and can't make it into the clinic. Or at least that is the story I was given. I soon learned that she had been confined to her powered wheelchair for some time, and the broken leg just made it more difficult to transfer into and out of the chair. She had been managing, and then with one small broken bone, suddenly was not managing at all.

I enter the house, noting the inevitable drawn shades, the clutter and piles of just pure stuff everywhere, the nick marks and gouges on all the door jambs from the wheelchair's tortuous path. Barbara's daughter fills the room with her personality and size. She is herself parked on the couch by the door, presiding over the scene with a cigarette perched on her lower lip. Barbara waits on her powered chair, immobile in its turning radius, the only clear area between the kitchen and the living area. She waits, trying occasionally to get a word in over her daughter's torrential output. Barbara is nearly deaf, had a hearing aid which cannot be located now, or was broken but then lost, or perhaps it was the fault of the dealer representative who failed to return a phone call. She cannot hear, does not follow the conversation and so knowing when to try to interrupt becomes impossible. She is a small woman, and getting smaller. Emaciated almost, her skin stretched on her arms, legs and chest then all folded up on her face into furrows and creases of worry and pain. She has no teeth and I have no time today for the convoluted story from her daughter of what happened to her dentures. Her right lower leg is encased in a plastic immobilizer. Somehow, she manages to be remarkably adept at maneuvering the joystick on the wheelchair and turns to face me.

Barbara's medical history is daunting, with surgeries, procedures, specialists, lists of drugs, "lost to follow up" here and there, consultations with social workers and every ancillary service that modern medicine has created: home health, physical therapy, dietician, case management, etc. And after reading pages of records, I compare that to the person seated in front of me, in her home. The written documents are vastly over-determined. She cannot even locate her pill bottles, and certainly cannot relate to anything documented in her records. She is worried about pain, and that no food tastes good.

This is only my second visit to Barbara's house. Her primary care physician -- PCP -- asked me to take over care as the patient kept missing appointments at the clinic. Her primary care clinic participated in a relatively new Medicare program called "Medical Home". This is an initiative sponsored by primary care organizations to better connect patients to their providers and clinics. The idea is that modern patients negotiate a complex system, and although much of the care is provided by specialists, benefitting from the system requires a more permanent spot where the patient is known in more depth, and can be helped with more than just pills, but social services, behavioral services and such. The medical home is a recognition of what every patient has known for years: our medical system is not very "homey". I hope the initiative is working for some patients, to help them feel more at home in our system, and increase their trust in it. For people like Barbara, the glaring hole in the medical home is the lack of the physical home. Barbara's medical home offered a suite of theoretical services, none of which were actually helping her, and none of which reflected her values as manifested in her dingy, cluttered, and utterly priceless space on this earth.

Today, I am visiting with a social worker from Adult Protective Services. After Barbara fell out of her wheelchair -- causing the leg fracture currently encased in a brace -- the hospital felt compelled to report her living situation to the state. Healthcare workers, and many other social service professions, are required to report suspected abuse, of both children and adults, primarily elders. The state then makes a comprehensive assessment, visits, interviews those involved, and determines whether the individual is safe or requires a state intervention to remove them to a safer situation. I don't envy these representatives of government who attempt to apply some sort of objective standard of safety to the chaos of real people's lives. They can't win of course. When they don't act and something terrible happens, they are castigated in the media and by politicians. When they do act and use the power of the state to remove people from their homes and families, a different segment of the population excoriates them. Mostly my job is to help keep people in their homes when they want to be there. Today I am supposed to help in this quasi-divine assessment of what the future holds for Barbara.

Precisely one day after my first visit here, I got a phone call from the emergency room that Barbara had fallen out of her chair again and now fractured the other leg. She was in the hospital for a consult with the orthopedic surgeon to determine whether she would benefit from a surgery to set the bone and screw it together. She has severe vascular disease, clogged arteries going from the heart down to the legs, so her healing capacity in the legs will be limited. Any surgery there risks the wound not knitting together and instead opening up, requiring more procedures and usually ending in amputation of the leg itself. And yet without hardware to hold the bones, she will be in pain, and able to move even less than before. I sigh as I think of the upcoming Adult Protective Services visit; surely this is the sort of danger that our society is trying to prevent with its protection programs. But perhaps, with all this pain, this time Barbara will agree to move to a rehabilitation facility for a while?

Down the hallway, in a small room with a low mattress, we maneuver into Barbara's bedroom. "Show me how you transfer from the chair to the bed," I ask. The diminutive act of moving the body from one position to the next often defines a person's ability to live in certain settings. Can she get from bed to a commode to a chair? And how much assistance is required? Can her dysfunctional daughter, her companion in this misfit household, maneuver between the dresser and the bed and the power wheelchair, stabilizing Barbara as she awkwardly pivots on the plastic splint on her leg?

Ominously previewing the scene, my imagination fails to see how this danse macabre will play out, day after day, without a catastrophic tumble of fragile limbs and full commodes.

"We have a caregiver every day," her daughter inevitably pipes in from the other room through her dangling cigarette. "She's the one that moves her."

The caregiver, paid through her disability benefits, does seem competent. But she leaves at 5pm. And does not come on the weekends. If you squint and hope, this situation could almost work, unless you focus on the cracks and gaps like what happens when she has to go to the bathroom at 1am. For the medical world where I work, "Discharge to home" becomes a phrase for a disposition, the final order before washing the hands. For patients, the phrase means "get out of jail" and restart real life. Recommending to Adult Protective Services that this home simply is not medically safe is likely the rationally correct thing to do. But my culture has forcefully moved so many people from their homes over the centuries, all for so-called rational reasons. Some sort of twisted racial memory overwhelms me as I negotiate the dark battered hallway lined by shelves of canned soup and candy, knocking over ashtrays next to the peeling drywall. This is a crazy house and a crazy dangerous home, and a medical or social disaster is likely to occur at any moment, but it's Barbara's crazy home, and her one goal in life is to live there, day by day, in shades-drawn semi-darkness and physical pain. So we make some plans, tweak a medication, and agree to keep assessing the situation. I leave the social worker on the sidewalk as we get back in our vehicles.

Inevitably I get the call the next day from the hospital where she has arrived after being brought by ambulance after falling out of her chair. Her left leg now has the same fracture as the right. The doctor is calling me because she is worried about sending her home again with two broken legs. It's all so predictable sometimes, like one of our favorite stories that we just keep reading over and over. Barbara's daughter has an explanation for what happened. "We know now what not to do and that won't happen again," she implausibly claims.

Every Ending has a Story

"Rashid, meanwhile, was arguing with Snooty Buttoo. 'Surely you don't want me to tell just sugar-and-spice tales?' he protested. 'Not all good stories are of that type. People can delight in the saddest of sob-stuff, as long as they find it beautiful.'" -- Salman Rushdie, Haroun and the Sea of Stories

America, as a primarily immigrant nation, is characterized by our ancestors having left their homes. Here out in the far West, at the end of the Oregon Trail, we remain the closest to this foundational history. In some sense, the leaving of the home, striking out on the adventure, the exploration, and the colonization, all define our Western civilisation. Having left the home, we have spent generations trying to find, or create it, again. Not only did our ancestors leave their homes, they imagined their new one as a scene of struggle. The mythic homesteader wresting a living from untamed wilderness dominates our interactions with our physical environment. The harsh Western geography and climate exacerbated this tendency. Those of us who inherit this ethos tend to trust in technological fixes to manipulate our inadequate or hostile surroundings.

Medicine participates in this cultural struggle over the loss of the home, and the faith in environmental manipulation to create human well-being. Every time we leave our house for the doctor's office, we have a hard time returning "home", for we are overtaken, in some small way, by a foreign medical structure and ideology that saves us, preserves us, carves on our bodies, and changes the places we can physically exist. Can I help Barbara to make it work in her home with now two broken legs? Somehow a disabled old woman with two broken legs and a dysfunctional daughter, trying to make a home in a darkened house cut off from their neighbors and social structures, encapsulates why our health care does not work well either. And why home visits are needed, and why a reimagination of health is needed, and why neither will happen until we find we find something authentic and local everywhere.

Our medical system will only reflect the care we want, in the communities we want, if we somehow come to terms with what Americans mean by coming home. Mrs. J, with her progressive lung disease and difficulties breathing, encapsulates the terrible inertia in the human condition toward always choosing another treatment. Bodily suffering and decay, or even the prospect of it, push nearly all of us to say "yes" to whatever new treatment or drug is on offer. It requires a compelling counter narrative of acceptance such as Joe and his wife found in their tiny RV, a proud symbol not only of their poverty, but of their freedom. Michael religiously attended all his subspecialist appointments where each particular organ was tallied and treated. But he never improved. "He" never improved as an integrated being because what is good for one system can be harmful to another. The body is layered and connected, in ways that our health system is not.

Those who stay home, who cultivate a home, admit that they have a destiny which is imposed upon them. They have things they accept rather than fight. The homesteader spends their time battling the environment, while the native spends their time adapting themselves to it. Western medicine encourages a homesteading mentality towards health. Mr. S saw his body as a collection of increasingly cheap parts that had simply failed and needed replacing. If we pay more, we can buy better quality parts next time.

Health represents the very fabric of our space-time, as Mrs. J finds when her lung disease makes even the act of breathing an effort. I am not optimistic that health care as a free market will deliver better human lives. The market will work as it always does, delivering more parts more efficiently. And there may be some areas where that is desirable even. But more parts will not show us the path for graceful acceptance of our mortal coil.

The consequences of our faith in manipulating our environment is coming home to roost as the climate warms and natural ecosystems require ever greater human input to be "managed". So too goes our health. Where will we find the balance between technological preservation of human life and acceptance of human mortality in graceful, culturally informed ways?

Recently, the giant enterprise of the industrial-medical complex has made progress. We now have palliative care, which brings back the focus to patient interactions, and really listening to what is important to patients. And we have "medical homes". And we have patient-centered care. These terms point to how the system is slowly changing, yet they often point out how far we have to go as well. How could there be any other type of medical care except "patient-centered"? The very existence of this term highlights the problem, that our care has not even been patient-centered. And patient-centered itself really only gets us halfway, because it still defines a person as a patient, and we should be providing human-centered care, where health is part of being human rather than a separate system, with its own routines and goals. The creation of health as a separate economic sphere has created our tendency to regard our bodies as machines, complaining of the cheaply made parts when we get sick or simply age.

Access to improved hygiene, diet and basic medical care has improved life spans everywhere. Consequently, more people are living with chronic diseases, and more people are becoming "poly-chronic", that is, they have multiple overlapping chronic diseases. Routine medical care such as minor infections, gallbladder surgery and broken limbs has become protocolized, safe, and routine. Within the limits of what medical science knows how to do, routine care should become as safe as airline travel. And the boundaries of what has become routine for medicine are astounding and ever-growing. Genetic manipulations, artificial organs, and biological pharmaceuticals will expand the lives that can be saved exponentially. We will all become patch-work creatures held together by technological marvels. And those of us who have been cured and saved multiple times by "routine" high-tech medical care, will subsequently become medically complex and require an entirely different type of system. We will all be monsters soon, let loose upon the world without proper thought as to how to be a constructed human rather than a natural one.

Creating a home for Frankenstein's progeny will require a new mode for medicine quite unlike the old. The new medicine will have to go block by block, and be high-touch rather then high-tech. The new medicine won't be provided exclusively by doctors, but by a multidisciplinary team that does not so much *cure* as re-connect. The monster is lonely, has no name, and is driven from polite society. We risk duplicating that terrible error over and over throughout our cities and countryside. Complex medical care means learning to live with, and live well with; it means suffering with, and coming to terms with. Complex care requires confronting the past, both the history of the medical system, and the cultural past that leads up to each patient's current situation.

Our country has to face the fact that we have never really had a "system" for health, but instead we have believed that individuals simply make free choices, and then must live with the consequences. However, there may be no such thing as a "free" choice with health. Poverty, limited access, culture, history, and educational disparities constrain choices before they can even be conceived. People do not consume healthcare so much as are consumed by it. The idea that people can make health decisions like they choose refrigerators is laughable to those of us who really engage with patients. Endless choices only lead to endless unhinged monsters, roaming the world, running up medical bills. Equally, we do not yet understand how to hold individuals accountable for the gamut of daily choices that they do have access to, and make. We can expect more self-agency from patients. We will likely find that self-agency cannot be taught or cajoled, but it can be mentored. Care in the home forces patients to confront their personal situations and health goals in a way that visits to facilities, where one is just a consumer in a health transaction, do not. Sitting at your kitchen table feels real; sitting in a clinic lobby feels like shopping.

Humanity has never before confronted complex chronic medical care. Complex chronic people simply died. So now we are facing the consequences of our own medical successes and societal failures. As culture has disintegrated, medicine has been tasked with stepping in and fixing diets, loneliness, destructive choices, and systematic discrimination. Somehow, it just might be possible.

While driving home I get a report that Tom has been admitted to the hospital, again. Despite my visits and despite our whole care-team. It will be an expensive stay. And he will feel belittled and maligned and get angry at the whole medical world again. Did something more serious happen? I wonder, or did we just not create enough trust in our last visit there, so he felt abandoned and called the ambulance? It's a puzzle.

"So what's the story?" I ask over the phone. Did he smoke too much marijuana and start vomiting? Or, has he been finding some narcotics on the side and is now withdrawing from them? Or will his abnormal lab actually turn into a real cancer and we will find carcinoid this time? The perplexing cases are always a motivation. Doctors try to simplify complex signs and symptoms by assigning labels, which we then call “diagnoses”. But the reality is that we love puzzles. We want to be mystified. The clouds seem to lift over the west hills in the distance, and the traffic moves more quickly.

This enigma will await me tomorrow. For now I get to arrive home and greet my family, and son, who is sitting peacefully and waiting, waiting for a walk, waiting for a word, and perhaps a quiet moment on the couch. Has he had a seizure today? Has he eaten well, or perhaps had a disastrous day with multiple seizures and vomiting, and now lies semi-conscious in a post-ictal state? The complexities of illness are overwhelming.

Loss and sadness seem to define the human condition and I have become a specialist in watching disease take away freedom. The arts and literature are the human creations that allow us to celebrate loss, sometimes as tragedy, sometimes as comedy. Patients need to see their medical histories in these larger contexts, and I need to see my work in the same way. Hope resides in the thought of the next patient; the one that I might help. The next one that will redeem me. I need the next encounter, the next twist and next turn, the unknown that awaits around the corner here on the street I know so well. I need to hear another patient story, another

"History of Present Illness". And I will need to make sense of that story by tapping into other stories of other people and places and times. I will "re-story" the patient's story and tell it back to her, sometimes substituting medical diagnoses for the symptoms that she tells me. And sometimes there will be no diagnosis, just tragic symptoms that no one understands, and those are the stories that require the larger human story. Literature, philosophy, and religion will absorb these accounts of powerlessness as we rage against our fate as humans. Re-living the patient's story as part of the human story will force me to keep feeling the personal impact of that illness, and so save me from the sterile burnout of the jaded caregiver. Humanism is the study of complexity, and it will be required for the complex patient, and me, the complex caregiver. I thought I was the medicine man, but I find that like everyone else, I am just another story addict.

Made in the USA
Las Vegas, NV
19 December 2022

63420508R00132